Cycling
Southeast Asia

Cycling
Southeast Asia

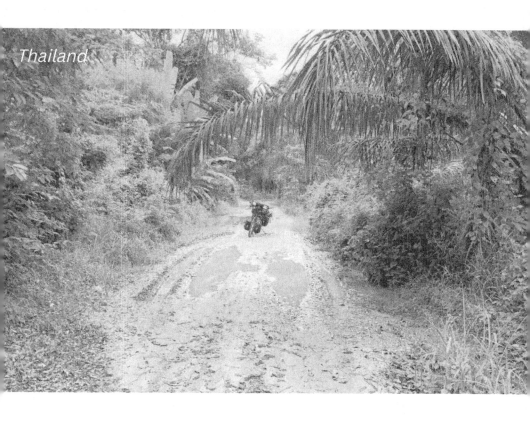

Thailand

John Peel

Content

Introduction

We recognise that cyclists possess unique preferences and requirements, so we provide extensive information on equipment, routes, visa regulations, phone connectivity, local cuisine, and other factors to help you optimise your cycling experience in this extraordinary part of the world. Moreover, this information can be applied to plan cycling excursions in other regions.

We do not wish to impose our recommendations on cyclists, as we, too, are enthusiastic cyclists who appreciate our personal preferences and individuality. As such, we respect the variety of cycling choices and encourage every cyclist to decide based on their preferences.

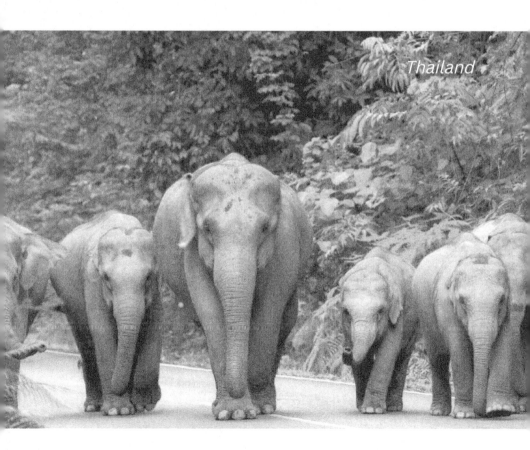

Thailand

CHAPTER ONE
Cycle & Gear

If your cycling journey is limited to Southeast Asia and not part of a more extensive world tour, it's advisable to pack as lightly as possible. Many travellers find that just two rear panniers and a bar bag are sufficient. Even bikepackers who are used to travelling light may be able to shed a few extra pounds. Cyclists using recumbents, tricycles, or other bike types often maximize available space.

The high temperatures, humidity, and damp conditions in Southeast Asia can be exhausting unless you're accustomed to them or reside in a region with similar weather patterns. Some cyclists prefer a fully loaded bike, packed with all their essential items and comforts for any situation.

Travelling light is essential in Southeast Asia due to the weather, but it's also practical because accommodations can be very affordable compared to Western standards. The cost of a popular campsite pitch in Europe can be comparable to that of a self-contained room with air conditioning, a shower, a TV, a bed, a refrigerator, Wi-Fi, and ample space to secure your bike and gear. Unless you're on the coast, staying in an air-conditioned room rather than a hot and humid tent on the frequently damp ground is preferable.

Although it's unlikely you struggle to find accommodation, having a super lightweight tent is still a good idea. An ideal tent would have a secure inner meshed area and a removable outer cover, perfect for hot and dry nights or stays inside the properties of locals, temples, huts or other shelters to keep out insects and other wildlife. Bivvy bags are acceptable in Southeast Asia but only suitable if you stay on the coast, with refreshing sea breezes and fewer insects and other creatures. Lightweight sleeping bags are fine, but synthetic materials are preferable to down, as the latter can retain moisture and be challenging to dry and clean in this climate. A pure silk sleeping bag liner is a simple and affordable option that many cyclists find comfortable and practical. The thin material provides warmth while keeping bugs at bay. A silk liner is also recommended while sleeping on beds in less-than-sanitary accommodations.

You might only require simple and lightweight cooking equipment to prepare a hot drink or a light meal of porridge or noodles. Since gas bottles may not be readily available for some stoves, multifuel stoves are a more practical option. If you're willing to explore street food or dine in small, locally-owned restaurants, you'll be delighted with the affordable and nourishing food options that abound in Southeast Asia.

A small water filter like a UV light pen or LifeStraw can prove helpful while occupying minimal space. While water is generally accessible, a filter will be beneficial if you have concerns about its safety.

You'll need a basic repair and maintenance kit. Although many bike shops or roadside mechanics in most places can assist you with nearly anything, it's still crucial to carry enough tools, replacement tubes, and even a foldable replacement tyre to ensure a safe and successful journey.

Prioritize waterproofing. Panniers and other bags should either be waterproof or equipped with waterproof covers since heavy, sometimes torrential downpours are frequent and can cause flooding on the roads. While you may be fortunate and experience minimal rainfall during your journey, it's best to be prepared. Wearing leggings and a heavy jacket is not recommended. Instead, a lightweight poncho with waist ties will suffice, preventing it from flapping in the wind or being pulled by passing vehicles.

A collapsible umbrella is popular among some riders, allowing them to seek temporary shelter underneath during sudden and heavy downpours while parked until the rain subsides.

It is recommended to bring credit and debit cards while travelling, and when using an ATM, try to use ones located in banks for added security. Additionally, inform your providers about your travel plans and the countries you will visit to prevent them from blocking your cards during use. Regarding safety, having a reliable mobile phone or two is also essential. Unlocked phones are handy as SIM cards are easily replaceable.

It is advisable to wear lightweight clothing as the sun can quickly burn the skin even on overcast days, so dressing appropriately and using sunscreen with a minimum SPF of 30 is recommended. A bandana or headband can be worn to keep the sweat out of your eyes, and a well-ventilated helmet will help keep your head cooler. Cycling gloves can provide a better grip if your hands become too sweaty. Additionally, a good pair of cycling sunglasses can protect your eyes from the sun's rays and debris on the road.

Having a basic first aid kit is crucial for any journey. Minor injuries like cuts and scrapes can quickly become infected in humid conditions, making it important to treat them promptly.

Cyclists tend to have strong preferences for their tyre brands and models. Choosing tyres less prone to punctures in Southeast Asia is essential, as changing or repairing inner tubes repeatedly in the heat and rain can be exhausting. Additionally, some regional roads can be harsh, so you may consider comfort when selecting tyres. Tyres with a width of at least 32mm (1.25 inches) up to 50mm (2 inches) or wider may be preferred depending on the terrain and the weight of your load. However, ensure that your bicycle can accommodate such wide tyres before choosing.

Many options are available when choosing a bike for your journey, including trikes, recumbents, touring, expedition, electric-assisted, etc.

However, if you're planning on using an electric-assisted bike, it's important to note that you will need to find campsites that have charging facilities available. These campsites are scarce in some areas, so it's essential to plan accordingly. Alternatively, electric-assisted bikes can be used for those planning on staying in rooms each night, as they are more readily available. Make sure to bring plug socket converters suitable for the regions you plan on visiting.

Expedition and mountain bikes are well-suited for off-road cycling in areas such as the hills and mountains of Laos, remote regions of Vietnam, and many roads away from main roads in Cambodia. However, it is worth noting that road conditions in Laos can be poor. Thailand has the best road conditions, followed by Vietnam, Cambodia, and Laos. For Thailand and Vietnam, a lightweight road touring bike would suffice, but conditions can be more demanding for Cambodia and Laos.

Bromptons and other smaller foldable bikes are suitable for cruising on many roads in Thailand and Vietnam. Not all roads in Cambodia and Laos are in poor condition, as many routes are still in excellent shape outside of town. However, the quality of roads in Cambodia and Laos is different from those of Thailand and Vietnam overall.

The optimal wheel size for the region is a topic of discussion and will depend on the cycling plan. When comparing spokes of equal quality and quantity, 26" wheels are better suited for off-road cycling as the spokes are shorter and can withstand rough terrain better. On the other hand, 700c wheels with hub gears will have shorter spokes in the rear.

Tourers in the region usually prefer travelling on tarmac or concrete roads with occasional gravel tracks, making 700c wheels an excellent choice. Most sizes of tires, particularly 700c or 26", are widely available in the area, with 700c being as easy to find, if not more so, compared to 26" wheels that were at one time much easier to locate. Tubes are also plentiful.

It's recommended to take a couple of spare spokes even if you can't true a wheel, as bike shops can usually do it for you but might not have your spoke size. Spokes take up very little space. Taking them along is a good idea.

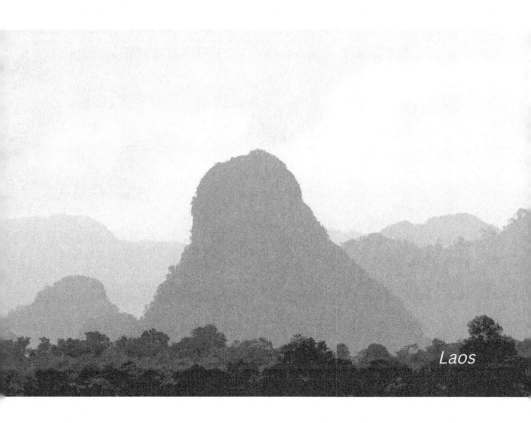

Laos

Any type of handlebar, such as butterfly bars, drops, or bulls, will suffice, but an upright position is recommended for a more comfortable ride while enjoying the scenery. As for the saddle, you can choose one you're accustomed to. For example, if you're sitting more upright and putting more weight on the saddle, opt for a wider, more comfortable one. On the other hand, if you're a lightweight rider leaning forward with more weight on the handlebars, a narrower saddle may suffice. However, touring is usually about comfort rather than speed, so it's essential to prioritize comfort over aesthetics when selecting a saddle. Saddle preferences are personal, so it's up to the individual.

Because of the frequent wet and humid conditions, cyclists often prefer disc brakes, particularly in hilly regions. Nevertheless, rubber brakes or disc brakes will do the job. Flat pedals are popular, primarily because of the weather, the laid-back style of travelling in the region and being able to wear comfortable footwear such as Crocs and sandals. However, the rain can cause rubber pedals to become slippery. Straps or clips may be helpful.

CHAPTER TWO
Navigation, SIMs, & Electricity

Navigating your way around these regions is straightforward. You only need a data sim card (SIM) and a smartphone. Those who use Garmin and other branded GPS navigation devices with preloaded maps and software will be fine, too. Communicating with local people can often take time and effort. As strange as this might sound, in some areas, even if you can say a few words in the local language, many out-of-the-way villagers might not get past the fact that you are a tourist and will not seem to understand what you are saying. Smartphones can use considerable power, so keeping a charge is essential. In addition, the phone will come in handy to locate food shops and restaurants, places to stay, and other essential services.

While solar panels and dynamo wheel hubs are popular among cyclists, battery banks are more cost-effective and convenient if you stay in budget accommodations. These banks are easy to charge in your room, and compact versions can provide power for several days on a single charge. Additionally, you can use them to charge other devices, such as Bluetooth speakers and cameras. Remember to obtain the appropriate socket adapters for the power outlets in the country you are visiting.

We recommend bringing a high-quality universal adapter that can be used with various outlet types across all these regions. Remember that a travel adapter only enables you to connect your devices to a different outlet physically and does not modify the voltage or power supply frequency.

- Type A - Mostly used in the US, Canada, Mexico, Central America, China and Japan. No other plug types will fit in an A outlet.
- Type B - Similar to type A, but with an extra pin for grounding. They are mainly used in the US, Canada, Mexico, Central America and Japan. Plugs of type A will also fit into a type B socket.
- Type C - The standard European plug. They are commonly used in Europe, South America and Asia, but in several other countries. Type E and F Plugs will also fit in a type C outlet.
- Type E - Mainly used in France, Belgium, Poland, Slovakia and the Czech Republic. Plug types C and F also fit in a type E outlet.
- Type F - Used in almost all European countries and Russia and is known as the Schuko plug. Type C and E Plugs will also fit in a type F socket.
- Type G - From British origin, mainly used in the United Kingdom, Ireland, Malta, Malaysia and Singapore, but in several other countries. No additional plug types fit into an outlet of type G.
- Type O - Used exclusively in Thailand. Plugs of type C will also fit into a type O socket, and there is unsafe compatibility with type E and F plugs.

Power Sockets in Thailand

The commonly used power outlets in these regions are compatible with parallel flat prongs (US/Japan) or two round pins, so it's recommended to bring adapters for both types. Some hotels in the area also have three-pin sockets installed to cater to European visitors. Thailand utilises multiple outlet types, including A, B, C, G, and O. If your equipment requires grounding, consider using a dedicated type O adapter. However, standard adapters have generally avoided any problems. The voltage in this region is typically 220v, and the frequency is 50hz.

Power Sockets in Laos

Laos power outlets and plugs of types A, B, C, E & F. You can use equipment with adaptors if your country's voltage is 220V-240V. Most of Europe, Australia, the United Kingdom, Africa and Asia. Typically: Voltage - 230v. Frequency - 50hz.

Power Sockets in Vietnam

Vietnam power outlets and plugs, types A, B, C, D & G. You can use equipment with adaptors if your country's voltage is 220V-240V. Most of Europe, Australia, the United Kingdom, Africa and Asia. Typically: Voltage - 220v. Frequency - 50hz.

Power Sockets in Cambodia

Vietnam power outlets and plugs are types A, C, & G. You can use equipment with adaptors if your country's voltage is 220V-240V. Most of Europe, Australia, the United Kingdom, Africa and Asia. Typically: Voltage - 230v. Frequency - 50hz.

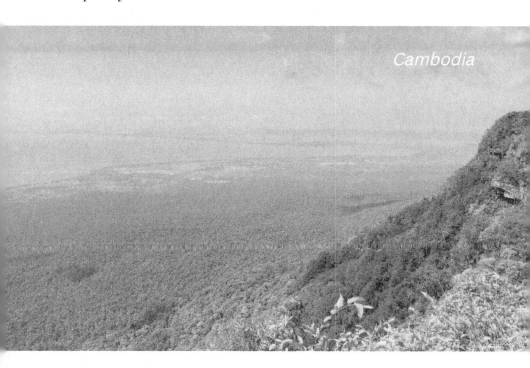

Cambodia

Obtaining a SIM is a straightforward process. You can purchase a data-only SIM in most small villages and towns without hassle. Some places offer SIMs with phone call minutes, which may require you to complete forms or provide personal information. Many smaller outlets may need to be equipped to handle those legal requirements. However, some data-only SIMs may come with a limited number of emergency minutes, which can often be topped up with a little effort.

You may be surprised at how inexpensive SIMs are compared to Western countries. You can get enough data for just a few dollars to last a month. While you may struggle to get a signal in some parts of the West, you may be pleasantly surprised at the excellent coverage of some networks in Southeast Asia.

Going to the SIM provider with the longest queue is recommended when beginning your tour and arriving at an airport. Although it may not always be the best option, it often is, so waiting a little longer is worthwhile. The provider will most likely install and activate the SIM for you.

If feasible, opt for unlimited data to have sufficient data to plan your routes and search for points of interest before or after a day's ride. With unlimited data, you can also call home and update your posts and blogs using social media services. Some cyclists prefer to use shareable tracking apps, such as WhatsApp, to track their daily activities with family and friends. If you bring a laptop, you can tether your phone to it for video and image editing or to download and watch movies. When cycling, solo tourers especially appreciate a few creature comforts.

It's a good idea to carry paper maps as a backup. Getting directions can be challenging in areas where you need more data or access GPS.

Many seek a unique experience, which includes inexpensive food and guesthouses, favourable weather, and thrilling adventures.

Thailand, Cambodia, and Vietnam are remarkable destinations that are generally safe. However, Laos is primarily underdeveloped, with many hilly areas. Finding villages with shops and accommodations can be challenging. Travelling along the Mekong River on the Laos side provides more options for food, water, and places to stay.

Cambodia, compared to some of its neighbouring countries, may have low levels of development. However, cyclists can still find plenty of places to stay and obtain food, water, and SIMs. Purchasing a SIM may be only slightly more challenging in Laos. To avoid any complications, it is recommended that you let the retailer set up the SIM card for you. The process should be quick and hassle-free.

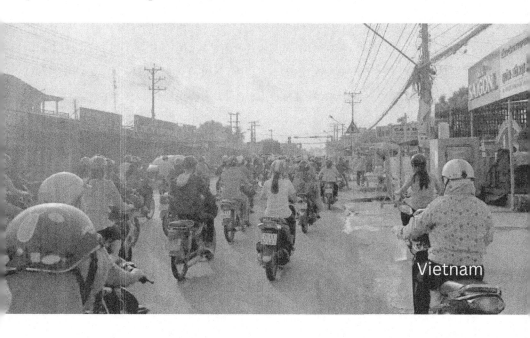

Vietnam

Regrettably, unrestricted data rates are frequently less swift than a predetermined data limit. Unlimited data may come at the expense of the highest speeds. So, a fixed data allowance is preferable if you require the highest speeds for downloading applications, sharing recorded content, or creating live videos. Additionally, if you deplete your data, you may not be able to top up, and obtaining a new SIM may be necessary.

Some tourists in Laos and Cambodia typically buy multiple SIMs from various providers. One SIM may not have coverage in certain areas, and temporarily switching to another can often resolve the issue. However, you should anticipate network congestion in some larger cities.

The region has a significant number of map applications. While Google Earth is an excellent app, there may be better options for navigation. Nevertheless, with Google Earth, you can often preview your destination and acquire a three-dimensional perspective of any obstructions, such as uneven terrain, dense foliage, and road conditions.

Visitors to these regions frequently follow well-trodden paths. Thailand is the most sought-after for established routes, offering excellent road conditions. Cyclists often travel along the coast towards Phuket or Krabi or head up to Chiang Mai or towards the border with Cambodia toward Siem Reap. However, for the more curious, the Korat Plateau in the northeast Isan region provides an incredible tour, allowing you to stray from the popular routes and explore the breadbasket of Thailand. This route will take you near the mighty Mekong and in proximity to the Laos border.

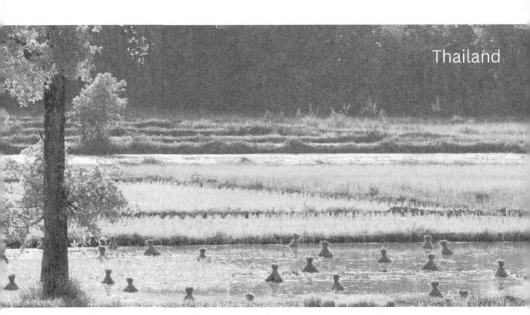

Thailand

DRAWING

CHAPTER THREE
Border Crossings

Depending on your country of origin and passport details, it can be relatively easy for cyclists to locate and cross borders in the region.

When crossing a border on a bicycle, it is reasonable that you may not have booked a return flight or arranged alternative transportation. Typically, border guards and personnel know this often do not require proof of onward travel or alternative transport.

Ensuring your passport has at least six months of validity remaining is recommended. Short periods on passports are viewed unfavourably and can raise suspicion that you have no intention of leaving.

While there have been instances of border-crossing staff scamming people, these occurrences are rare. In general, border personnel are friendly and helpful. Although the amount of money lost in these scams is typically not significant, it can be enough to make some people lose their temper and create a scene, which is understandable. However, if you suspect that you have been scammed and the amount is minimal, it is often better to let it go and focus on crossing the border smoothly.

The guards at each border come from distinct cultures, legal systems, ideologies, religions, and systems. For instance, Thailand operates as a constitutional monarchy, while Laos sees itself as socialist.

embracing communism, known as the Democratic Republic. As you cross the border from either country, you will notice a significant difference between the two nations, including the border guards and staff, who may seem distinct, but not necessarily in a negative way. It's crucial not to feel that you're being mistreated on one side versus the other, even if that's the case, since each country has its unique way of doing things.

"Border Bouncing" refers to crossing a border to obtain another visa for re-entry. Digital nomads often use this strategy to extend their stay in a particular country for several months or even years. Cycle tourists may also use this technique when their visa is about to expire, but they still wish to explore a specific country.

It is worth noting that crossing a border to obtain a visa as quickly as possible, even on the same day in some instances, is becoming less common. If you are not cautious, your visa application may be denied. Spending at least the best part of a week or more on the other side of the border is advisable before applying for a return visa.

Border crossings are often bustling with activity, with a daily influx of tourists arriving by coach, commercial vehicles, buses, and individuals visiting family or working in a neighbouring country. While there is no perfect time to plan your border crossing, mid-morning is typically the quietest at many crossings. Early morning or mid-afternoon tends to be busy, as people rush to work or try to beat the potential long lines. During lunchtime, many individuals believe that they will have given the early morning rush enough time to pass. In the evening, those who visited worked or went on day trips usually return. However, it's important to note that it can often be hit-or-miss depending on the border crossing.

Although there are over 20 land border crossings around Thailand, we will discuss a few that cyclists often use.

We have also included a brief description of a cross-sea border crossing located at the southwestern most point of Thailand, as it leads into one of the most sought-after regions in Thailand for tourists and visitors.

Tourists may be required to provide proof of their onward destination, such as a hotel reservation or booking. In such cases, it is recommended to spend the night near the crossing, make a reservation as proof of departure, and return to the checkpoint armed with the booking details. Alternatively, a person could use their mobile device to reserve accommodation while still at the checkpoint.

The reason why visa costs are not included is that they tend to fluctuate frequently—verifying if visas are obtainable upon arrival and the applicable fees before heading to each crossing is crucial. Given that circumstances may vary, it is advisable to stay updated to avoid wasting time and effort.

Make sure to verify the dates on the newly issued visa or visa stamp to ensure that the requested duration of the visa is accurate. If the visa duration is longer than requested, everything is fine. However, if it is shorter, correcting it before leaving the desk is crucial. This mistake is more prevalent than one might assume.

It is advisable to carry additional passport-sized photos as they can be helpful in various situations. For example, photographs may be required at certain border crossings, and there could be a possibility of charging extra fees for this service. Additionally, if there are variations in passport or visa photo sizes in different countries, it is recommended to carry multiple sizes. This foresight could save both time and money.

Thailand

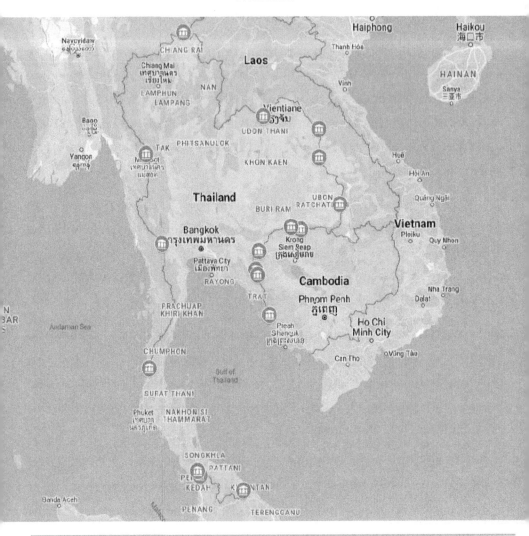

Thailand - South with Malaysia

Su-Ngai Kolok / Rantau Panjang

One of the reasons why this border crossing is popular between Thailand and Malaysia is the abundance of public transportation and amenities available in the area. There are several affordable accommodation options and stores where you can purchase the necessary items for your journey.

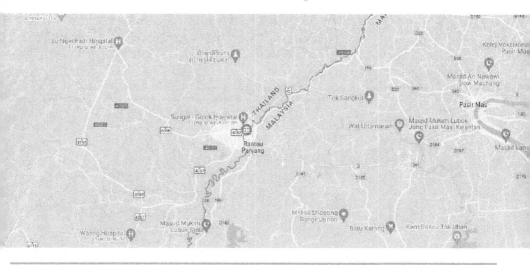

Sadao / Bukit Kayu Hitam

This is a less used crossing for tourists but one open 24 hours most days. Facilities are more plentiful on the Thailand side.

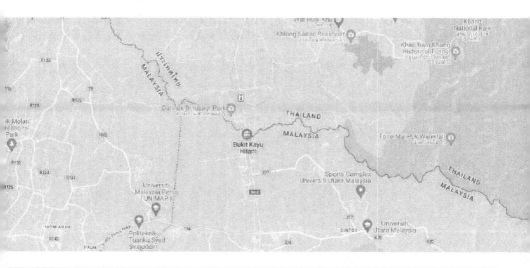

Padang Besar

This crossing is known to request proof of leaving Thailand before permitting entry. Not often, but it could be enough to cause issues at the border.

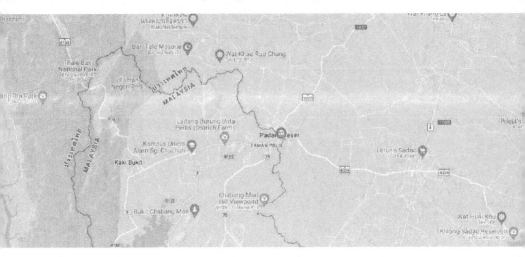

North and West with Myanmar

Ranong / Kawthoung

A half-hour-long boat ride can ferry cyclists between Thailand and
Myanmar. This region is stunning, with many famous, well-known islands
nearby.

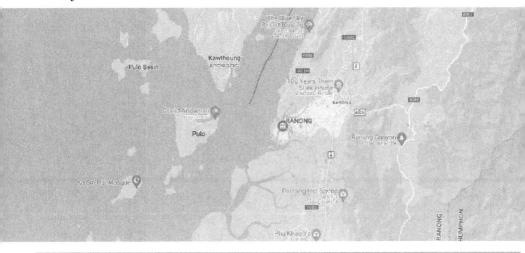

Ban Phu Nam Ron / Htee Khee

As of the time of writing, visas are not obtainable at this crossing. If you plan
to cross at this location, you must obtain your visa in advance, which many
people do in Bangkok. Remember that circumstances can change at any
crossing, so it's advisable to check beforehand.

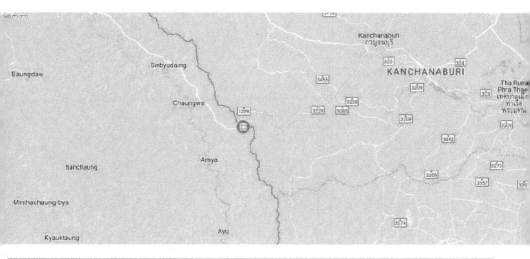

Mae Sot / Myawaddy

Similar to most border crossings with Myanmar, it is recommended to obtain your Myanmar visa beforehand to avoid potential issues that may arise. However, many individuals still manage to cross without any difficulties.

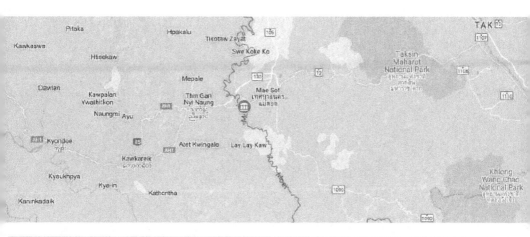

Mae Sai / Tachileik

This crossing is relatively remote. However, it is essential to note that many have been refused a crossing when border bouncing. The recommended approach is to spend at least one week on either side before attempting to re-enter the other.

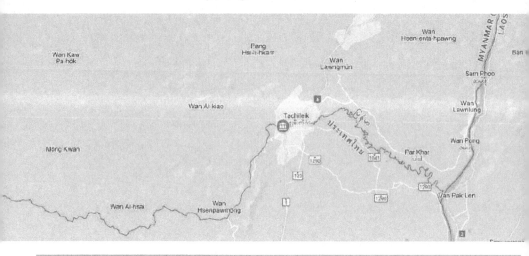

Thailand - East with Laos

Nong Khai / Vientiane

Crossing the Mekong River via the first Friendship Bridge is a delightful experience. There are numerous accommodation options, restaurants, and shops on the border. Nong Khai has a large ex-pat community and is well-established, while Vientiane, the capital city, is a vast sprawling metropolis.

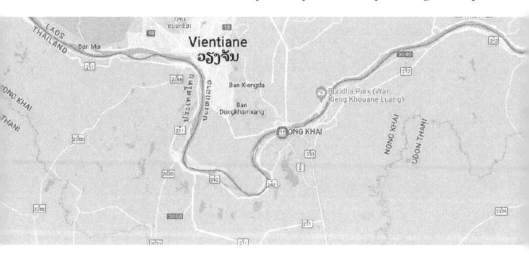

Nakhon Phanom / Khammouane

The third Friendship Bridge is located along a fantastic stretch. New smooth tarmac roads have been built along the Mekong River to Nakhon Phanom.

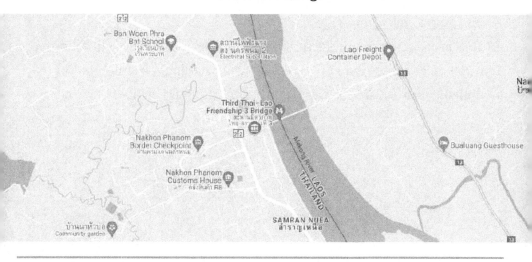

Mukdahan / Savannakhet

While riding alongside the Mekong River, you will encounter this border crossing and the second Friendship Bridge. The Thai side of the border boasts a relatively flat terrain compared to the hilly landscape of Laos. Some visitors have experienced lengthy visa processing times at this crossing. However, there are abundant accommodation options and numerous activities to keep you occupied. It's worth noting that the visa processing system was expected to improve from 2023 and beyond.

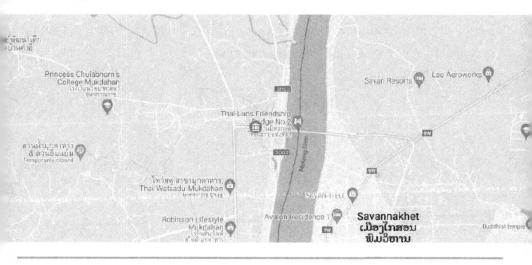

Chong Mek / VangTao

As this area is not a tourist destination, there are limited attractions or activities near the crossing. Therefore, while finding accommodation may be difficult, access to food, water, and supplies should be fine.

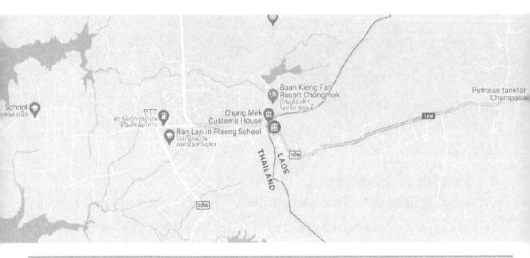

Thailand - South and East with Cambodia

Choam Sa Ngam / Anlong Veng

Despite its stunning scenery, Southeast Thailand attracts relatively few tourists, leaving the area relatively unexplored. On the Cambodian side, casinos are abundant and located close to the border, and there is a small town nearby where you can purchase supplies.

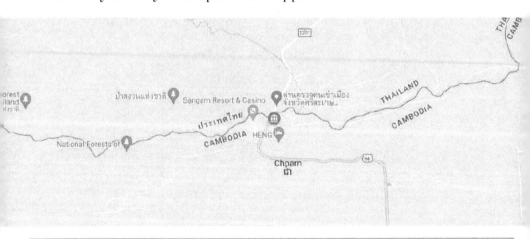

Border Crossings

Chong Jom / O Smach

This is a popular crossing. It approaches larger towns and major roads. When descending from Thailand's Korat Plateau to the lower lands of Cambodia, you will notice a significant difference in road conditions, vegetation, shops, and amenities, highlighting the height of the plateau. After Thailand, Cambodia may seem relatively impoverished, but its inhabitants are known for displaying the warmest smiles.

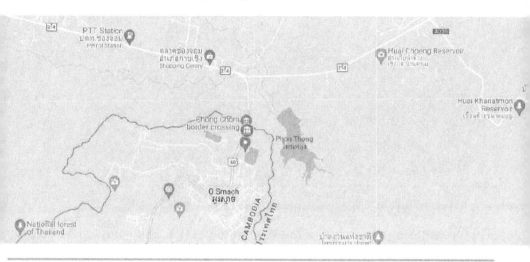

Aranyaprathet / Poipet

This border crossing can experience heavy traffic, with tourists travelling to see the Angkor Wat temple complex in Siem Reap, Cambodia, business travellers passing through, and those commuting between Bangkok and other destinations. However, from a cycling perspective, the main roads from Bangkok to Siem Reap, Cambodia and en route to Vietnam are mostly flattish, making for a more leisurely ride. Wind direction permitting.

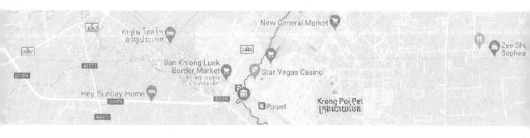

Ban Laem / Daun Lem

Compared to the busier Aranyaprathet / Poipet crossing located further north, this border crossing is quieter but still offers plenty of activity and finding supplies and guesthouses should be relatively easy from there.

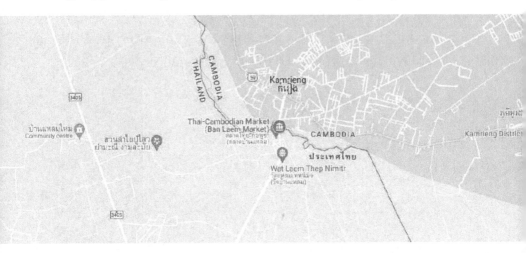

Ban Pakkad / Phsar Prum

This crossing is yet another minor one and not on a significant tourist route. However, you can still get a visa on arrival.

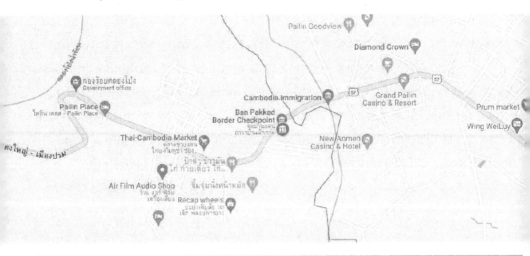

Ban Hat Lek / Cham Yeam

Located on the coastline between Cambodia and Thailand, this border crossing can experience high traffic. Acquiring a visa can feel like a lengthy process. Still, it can be an opportunity to take a break.

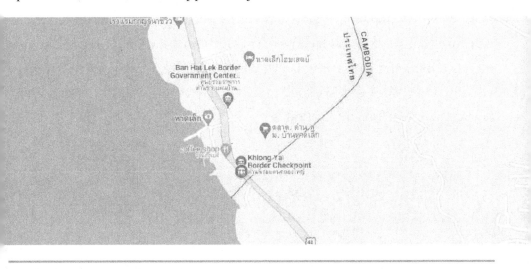

For crossings between Thailand and Cambodia, see Thailand crossings

Cambodia

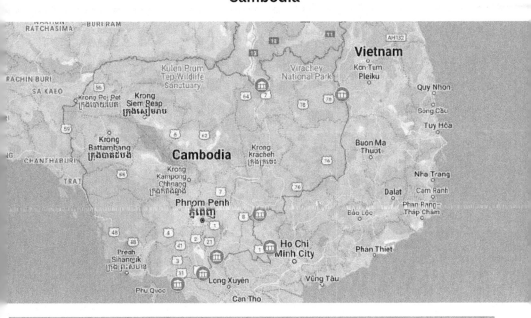

Cambodia - South and East with Vietnam

Bavet / Moc Bai

This one is the most frequently used among the border crossings between Cambodia and Vietnam, as it is situated along the major roads connecting Siem Reap, Phnom Penh, and Ho Chi Minh City. Furthermore, several nearby casinos in Cambodia attract visitors who are willing to spend some money. Obtaining a visa at this crossing is also the most straightforward. Usually, a two-week visa is issued unless you have an e-visa or another type of visa valid for a longer duration.

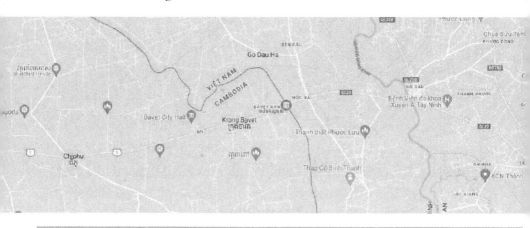

Vinh Xuong / Thuong Phuoc

This particular border crossing and the following two crossings are located near each other, with a distance of less than a day's ride. However, this crossing tends to be busier as it is one of the closest to Phnom Penh.

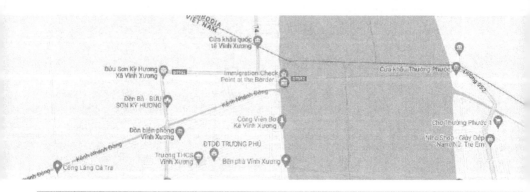

Phnom Den / Tinh Bien

This border crossing, located closer to the coast, is known for the abundance of motorcycle taxis vying for business with those crossing into Vietnam. However, as a cyclist, you won't have to contend with them, making it a good option. Crossing to Vietnam can be pretty chaotic compared to the calmness on the Cambodian side. Tuk-tuks are scarce, and the streets are filled with motorbikes and scooters.

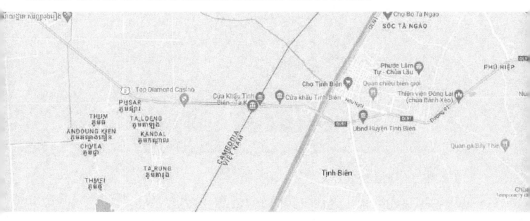

Ha Tien / Xa Xia

Located on the coast, this border crossing is perfect for cyclists exploring the coastal regions of Thailand, Cambodia, and Vietnam. There are more casinos on the Cambodian side, heavy traffic, and accommodation options.

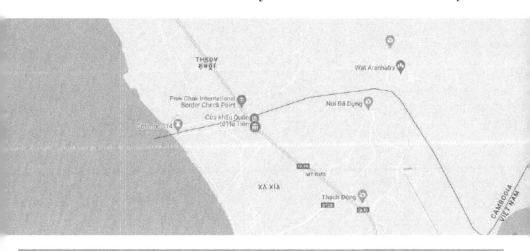

Trapang Thlong / Xa Mat

Farther north, this crossing was opened for tourists in 2007 and has become quite popular with motorcycle tourists.

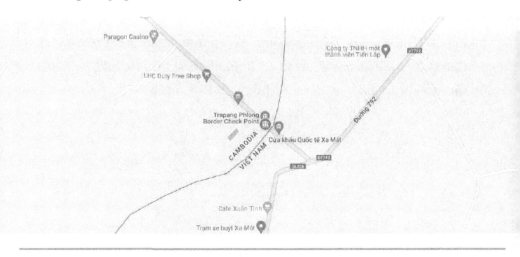

Oyadav / Le Thanh

This crossing is the final option for cyclists heading towards Vietnam from areas away from the coast or Phnom Penh. It is advisable to have an e-visa to avoid complications, as it can be quite a journey to reach this point. However, that may change, so do a little research beforehand, such as checking the opening times, fees, and necessary documents for crossing.

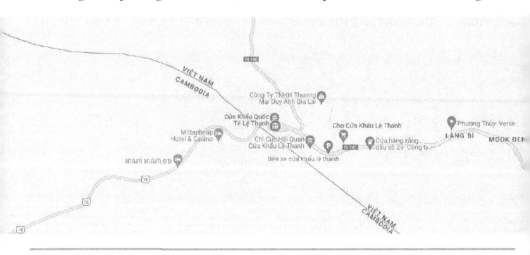

Cambodia - North with Laos

Tropaeng Kreal / Nong Nok Khiene

The only feasible option to cross from Cambodia to Laos is this crossing, which is about a week's ride from Phnom Penh. The journey to the border is long and thrilling, passing through the stunning "4000 Islands" region, where the Mekong River spreads into multiple tributaries and creates a unique landscape of islands. While the views are breathtaking, be prepared for dusty or muddy roads. As with other remote crossings, it's essential to check ahead and allow plenty of time to plan for the crossing.

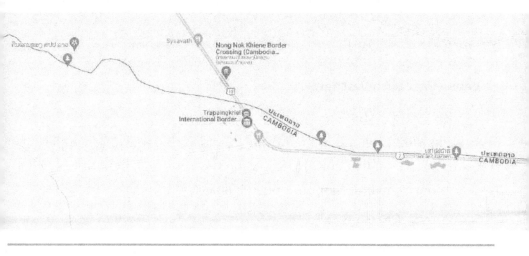

For crossings between Thailand, Cambodia and Laos, see Thailand and Cambodia crossings

Laos

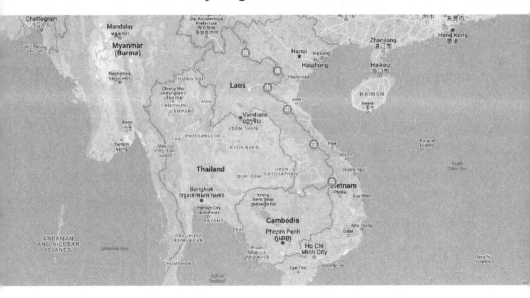

Laos - East with Vietnam

Bo Y / Ngoc Hoi

When entering from the Vietnam side, it's advisable to gather supplies as most shops are on that side. However, on the Laos side, item prices might be lower once you find shops or other facilities.

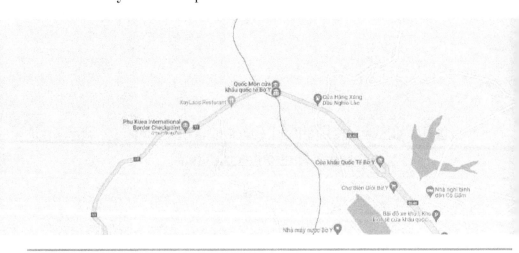

Nam Phao / Cau Treo

This crossing is similar to most overland crossings. Shops and places to stay are on both sides.

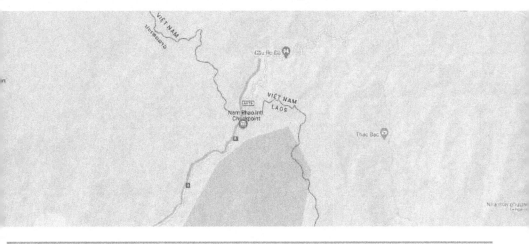

Dansavanh / Lau Bao

This border crossing is popular among travellers due to its reputation for being easy to pass through. However, it is essential to note that there are only a few shops and places to stay, primarily in Vietnam.

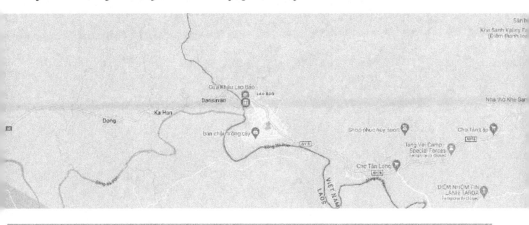

Sop Hun / Tay Trang

Due to the hilly terrain near this border crossing and the large towns on either side, it may be necessary to take a break and rest at a guesthouse. For those who plan to camp, it is essential to be cautious and select well-travelled areas or designated campsites, as Laos has a history of being heavily bombed, resulting in thousands of landmines and other weapons that still pose a risk to hundreds of people each year.

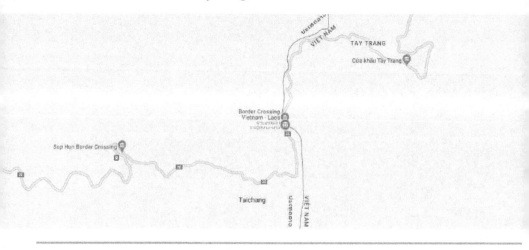

Na Maew (Na Meo) / Nam Xoi

Cyclists have found this crossing to be uncomplicated, with no issues encountered. Nonetheless, like other crossings, guards have asked for a dollar or two for no apparent reason. As a result, some cyclists pay the fee to expedite their crossing despite it being frustrating.

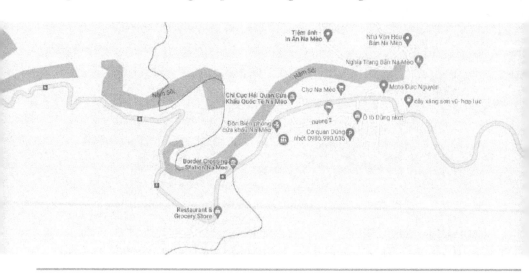

Nam Can / Nam Khan

This crossing is said to be in beautiful scenic surroundings. Compared to some, the border process is straightforward. However, expect some wet or foggy weather with the nearby hills holding onto clouds.

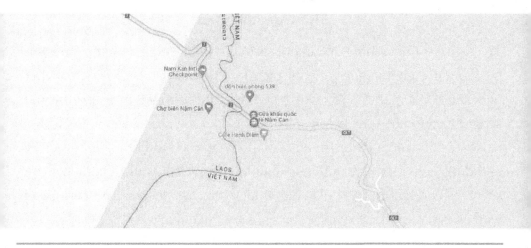

For crossings between Laos, Cambodia and Vietnam, see Laos and Cambodia crossings

Vietnam

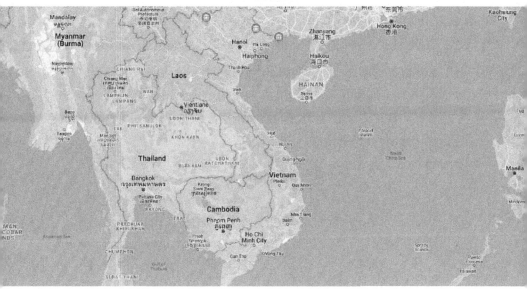

Vietnam - East with China

It is advisable to check the crossing regulations between Vietnam and China beforehand as they can be strict. There are three primary and popular crossings to the east: Mong Cai / Dongxing, Dong Dang / Ping Xian, and Lao Cai / Kekou.

Tips from the road

To ensure your essential documents are safe while you are on the road, it is best to make photocopies of your passport, driving license, visa, and other necessary documents before you leave. Keep these copies in a separate and secure location in your belongings. It's also an idea to leave copies with a trusted family member or friend back home in case you lose your originals and duplicates. Another option is to upload copies of your documents to a secure cloud-based drive or email folder for easy access. You can travel with peace of mind by having copies of your documents.

Southeast Asia is vulnerable to natural disasters and political instability from time to time, so it's important to allow ample time for touring and avoid having a schedule that's too tight.

Obtaining a doctor's note for prescribed medication before travelling to Southeast Asia is recommended, as certain drugs may be confiscated at border crossings. This includes items used in Testosterone Replacement Therapy and painkillers, sometimes considered recreational drugs. Failure to comply with regulations could result in fines or worse. Obtaining a doctor's note, which may require a small fee, will help ensure you can consume or use the medicines without issues.

NOTES

CHAPTER FOUR
On The Road In Southeast Asia

Thailand follows left-hand driving, while Laos, Cambodia, and Vietnam adopt right-hand driving, making it crucial to keep in mind while crossing their borders. Despite most vehicles adhering to their designated side, the situation can seem quite different on the road. Witnessing motorcycle commuters riding on any side they desire can be pretty unnerving.

The primary culprits for disregarding road rules are motorcyclists, who ride along the road's edge in the opposite direction, putting others in danger. Stand your ground in such situations. If you see another vehicle approaching you the wrong way, do not allow yourself to be pushed closer to the traffic when travelling the right way. Initially, this may cause anxiety, but eventually, it becomes second nature. Cyclists also ride on the wrong side, which is unsafe and not recommended.

Adapting to riding on the left or right may initially seem daunting If you are not accustomed to it, but in reality, it takes only a brief period to acclimate to the change. It's remarkable how quickly one can adjust.

In Southeast Asia, cycling two or more abreast or down the centre of a lane, which may be acceptable in your home country, can lead to severe consequences. It's advisable to use any available cycle lane, regardless of its rough appearance. On narrow, fast-moving roads with only a soft gravel shoulder, it's better to use it instead of the congested and hazardous tarmac. If cycling on the road's edge on gravel, ensure that you are as far over towards the verge as possible, allowing enough space in case of slipping on gravel. Additionally, the gravel shoulder may contain more obstacles, such as nails and glass, that can cause punctures, so it's essential to remain vigilant. Despite these challenges, the verge may still be the safer option for many.

In Southeast Asia, traffic tends to move smoothly and quickly, with frequent horn honking that is not typically aggressive. Horns often signal intentions, such as overtaking or expressing gratitude. In contrast, in some Western countries, drivers may harbour a strong dislike for cyclists, leading to aggressive honking and dangerous manoeuvres that can cause accidents. However, in Southeast Asia, cyclists generally do not experience this kind of animosity from drivers. Instead, vehicles tend to move together, yielding to each other and allowing for unpredictable behaviour. Because the traffic often moves like schooling fish, sudden turns or braking without reason should be avoided if possible. Other commuters may be only a few feet or less away on all sides and need help to react quickly. By gently moving with the traffic, cyclists can work harmoniously with drivers.

Opinions vary among cyclists regarding the prevalence of motorists driving under the influence of alcohol. Some believe that early mornings are the worst time for encountering drunk drivers, while others suggest that late nights and overnight hours are more dangerous. Regardless of the time, it is an issue that cyclists should consider. While cycling during the night is not recommended, many cyclists opt to ride at first light and finish before mid-afternoon due to the intense heat and humidity during the day.

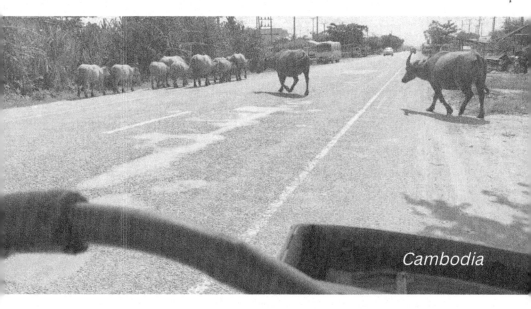

Cambodia

The phrase "When in Rome" emphasizes that road rules that apply at home may not be relevant in another country. However, most experienced drivers familiar with their country's highway code will adapt quickly. Others may require a bit more time, but only a little. It's important to research and understand the local road rules, regulations, customs, and cultural norms and to show respect for them. Even if you disagree with them, it's best not to express disapproval, as engaging in road rage arguments with strangers will only lead to negative outcomes. While you may feel capable of confronting one or two individuals, you may face an entire community that will come to their aid. It's better to move on or seek assistance from the police.

Staying hydrated is crucial when cycling in hot and humid conditions. In some cases, cyclists have fainted from heat exhaustion due to insufficient water intake and fallen onto the road. Water is widely available for purchase, but carrying extra bottles in emergencies is advisable. Despite the scenic beauty, the heat and humidity can make conditions intolerable for some cyclists, causing them to cut their trips short. While photos may depict lush greenery, they often fail to capture the actual intensity of the climate.

When cycling near coastlines, the cooler air from the sea can make the temperature more tolerable. The same applies to higher elevations, such as mountains and hilly regions. Conversely, lower areas, particularly those covered by forests or jungles, tend to be humid and hotter.

Cyclists may experience discomfort and illness from inhaling dust and toxins from passing vehicles. Dust can contain harmful substances from people, animal waste, and chemicals. Prolonged exposure to these pollutants can make cyclists feel sick and require a day or two of rest. Therefore, many cyclists are adopting a bandana or mask to cover their mouths while cycling, which has become increasingly popular. However, some may find it uncomfortable.

Certain regions anticipate encountering numerous potholes and poor road conditions. For example, Thailand's roads are predominantly well-maintained, followed by Vietnam, Cambodia, and Laos. However, traffic can be more frenzied in Vietnam due to the high volume of motorbikes.

The weather tends to be hot and humid, making many prefer starting and finishing their activities early. Opting to depart at dawn can be beneficial. The weather pattern can often involve relatively dry conditions during the first part of the day, with rain showers or storms arriving in the afternoon and often throughout the night, depending on the season.

Having insurance is crucial. In a worst-case scenario where you might find yourself severely injured thousands of miles away from home without insurance, your family may be obligated to cover hospital expenses or even repatriation fees getting you home. While obtaining insurance for a high-value cycle and gear can be challenging, acquiring coverage for injury, health, and certain types of theft, loss, and damage is often relatively straightforward. Numerous insurance providers offer such coverage, but it is essential to carefully review the fine print to ensure your requested coverage is included.

The frequency and severity of road flooding in Southeast Asia vary by region and season. Generally, many Southeast Asian countries experience a rainy season that lasts for several months, during which flooding is expected. In some areas, such as Bangkok, flooding is a regular occurrence during this season. In other regions, particularly coastal areas, flooding may occur due to tidal storm surges.

Road flooding can be hazardous for cyclists unfamiliar with an area or cycling conditions. The depth and speed of the floodwaters can be challenging to gauge. In addition, hidden hazards like debris, potholes, or damaged road surfaces may exist. Cyclists should stay informed about weather conditions and flood warnings in the areas they plan to visit. If flooding occurs, it is best to avoid cycling through floodwaters and to seek higher ground if possible.

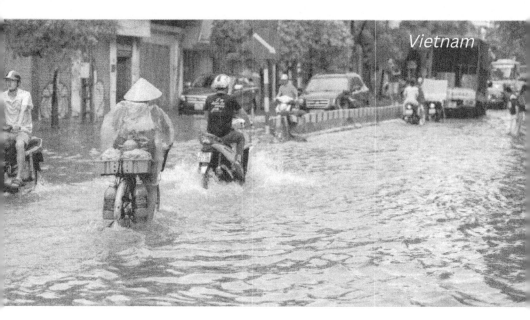
Vietnam

Eat to fuel your body. Even if you cycle mainly flat landscapes, the heat and humidity can be draining, so getting the proper nutrients is essential. Simple, highly nutritious foods are available hot or cold almost anywhere at very reasonable prices for most budgets.

Having a bad tummy can be challenging. While cycling, dealing with diarrhoea and finding a place to relieve oneself can be an unpleasant experience. Some people avoid consuming fish, including shellfish. Many regions' seafood and fish are farmed, and toxins and medications are commonly used to grow them. While many farms adhere to high standards, not all do, and consequently, the safety and healthfulness of the food produced can vary. Although coastal areas and big rivers such as the Mekong offer many edible fish species, pollutants can cause digestive problems in those unfamiliar with the local cuisine. Moreover, unfamiliar spices and other ingredients may also trigger gastrointestinal issues.

Consequently, if you experience digestive problems, it is advisable to refrain from drinking water for the day and instead consume plenty of non-diet carbonated drinks such as sports drinks, Sprite, or other fizzy beverages.

Additionally, avoid consuming ice that is not shaped like ice cubes. Often, roadside vendors chop ice from blocks using machetes or store it in chest freezers alongside canned goods and other food, sometimes raw fish and meat, which may compromise its safety and cleanliness.

Cycling from point A to B can be as simple as traversing a highway or major road network. However, while this approach allows you to cover a lot of ground, there is so much more to explore by taking a few detours every now and then. These detours don't have to be extensive; even a few miles away from the main road, everything can look vastly different. By taking these diversions, you could see the region uniquely and gain a deeper appreciation of the area.

Small towns and villages are a treasure trove of inexpensive, diverse food and drinks. Moreover, these areas are often less polluted with dust, mud, and fumes, providing a more pleasant cycling experience. Additionally, exploring these remote locations leads you to discover hidden gems such as temples or facilities where locals extend a warm welcome.

Exercise caution around the wildlife by ensuring your bags are tightly sealed and secure, as small critters may crawl inside or snakes may become entangled in your wheels. Monkeys may also attempt to snatch your belongings or become aggressive, while mosquitoes and other biting insects may emerge during the evening. Furthermore, be wary of larger creatures such as wild elephants and buffalo. Finally, to avoid heat buildup in your bags, it's best to open them several times throughout the day while keeping an eye on them.

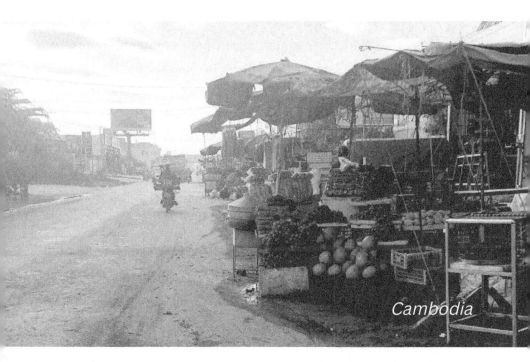

Cambodia

Border areas, particularly those between Myanmar, Thailand, Laos, Cambodia, and Vietnam, are known to have landmines and other unexploded weapons. Vietnam, for instance, has a landmine contamination rate of 20%, which has caused the deaths of thousands of individuals over the years. In addition, Cambodia and other regions are still grappling with landmine-related issues. Consequently, it's recommended that you stick to established routes and trails, especially when venturing off main roads, to minimize the risk of encountering such hazards.

Tour companies are active in many locations. A straightforward online search or inquiry on a forum can help you find a tour that perfectly meets your requirements if that style of travel is more to your liking.

Adjusting to the weather and any new cycle could be challenging if you're unaccustomed to the region's heat and humidity. So, getting acclimatised to the bike and learning how it performs under different conditions is best if you plan to bring a new bike to Southeast Asia. Familiarise yourself with basic repairs, such as changing a tire and tube, adjusting cables and other parts, and replacing brake pads or shoes. Additionally, inspecting the bike's nuts and bolts regularly is essential, as, in harsh road conditions, screws can loosen quickly. Similarly, it's beneficial to wear the clothing you plan to take before embarking on your trip to become accustomed to it. Even a few weeks of practice can make a big difference.

Avoid rushing, and take in as much of your surroundings as possible. Capture photographs and videos of the breathtaking scenery. Spending extra time documenting your journey will give you incredible images to cherish and share. Every mile or kilometre is a unique experience, and whether it's a challenging or easy day, it's a privilege many cannot afford or have time for. Unfortunately, not everyone will have the opportunity to embark on such a fantastic adventure. Hence, capturing high-quality footage and images during your tour is a must, as nothing is worse than regretting not having done so upon returning home.

Individual cyclists often interact more with local people than those cycling in groups or with a partner. Whether cycling alone or in a group, engaging with the locals and gaining insights into their cultures and customs is advisable. While most people you meet may be preoccupied with their work, some may attempt to sell you something during your interactions. However, it's essential not to feel bothered by their sales pitch but instead seize the opportunity to learn more about local attractions, restaurants, or accommodation options by spending a few minutes in their company.

Thailand is the most favourable for many cyclists of the four countries featured in this edition due to its superior road conditions, reasonable accommodation options, and numerous breathtaking islands and beaches to explore. Following Thailand, Cambodia is the next best option. While it may not be as affluent as Thailand or Vietnam, it boasts friendly locals, plenty of flat terrain, and notable tourist attractions such as Angkor Wat. Vietnam comes in third with its extensive coastline, resorts, bustling cities, and towns. The western and northern parts of Vietnam showcase stunning mountains and hilly landscapes. Conversely, Laos can be rugged in specific regions and appears less developed than the other three countries. However, it boasts stunning scenery, thick foliage, plenty of hills, and even a fast lowland waterway in the south.

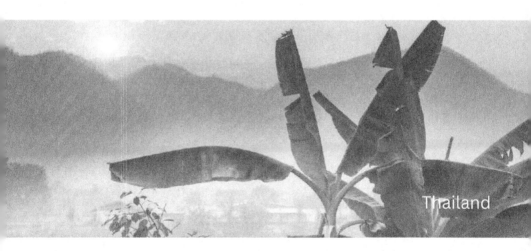

Thailand

Wearing a helmet is crucial. It helps maintain your safety. Additionally, the vents in the helmet help keep you cool as you cycle, which is particularly beneficial when riding in hot weather.

It's advisable to wear bright and reflective clothing while cycling in Southeast Asia to ensure that you are visible to other road users. The region experiences dark and overcast days for much of the year, with frequent heavy rainfall, making it challenging to spot cyclists not wearing reflective clothing. Being visible to others is crucial for your safety on the road.

A sturdy set of cycling sunglasses with durable lenses is essential to improve visibility against the sun's glare and shield your eyes from potential hazards such as stone chippings, dust, and other debris passing vehicles may kick up while riding.

As we have mentioned, storms can cause roads to flood, resulting in water levels reaching up to your pedals or even higher. To prepare for such situations, it is crucial to have reliable waterproof bags and clothing that can dry quickly.

Factor in rest days when cycling in hot and humid conditions, as the experience can be exhausting. Moreover, if you choose to spend your rest days in locations with exciting activities or serene environments, they can enhance the overall adventure of your trip.

Different from some parts of the world, many regions in Southeast Asia are less likely to want to barter the price of goods, particularly in rural areas, where language barriers may pose a challenge.

If you want to cycle on mostly even terrain, exploring central Thailand around Bangkok and onto the Khorat Plateau may suit you. While in Cambodia, the majority of the landscape is relatively flat. However, the northern part of the country can be undulating, and the Cardamom Mountains in the far south are rather large hills. Laos is the flattest in the country's southern region, while the remaining areas can be hilly. Southern Vietnam features some of the lowest lands in the country, such as the stunning Mekong Delta, characterized by numerous islands created by the tributaries of the Mekong River as it flows into the sea and is a joy to cycle.

CHAPTER FIVE

Safety & Security

Cycles and cycling gear are rarely stolen. However, when it does occur, it can abruptly end a tour, and seeking assistance from authorities or insurance companies can sometimes be difficult. Fortunately, bike theft, particularly cycles that appear expensive and complex and belong to cycle tourists or tourists in general, is not a common occurrence.

Southeast Asian thieves tend to target bags or smaller, easier-to-hide and sell items rather than expensive-looking cycles that will attract attention. It's unpleasant to admit, but in rare cases where a touring bike is stolen, it has been attributed to other cyclists or budget travellers. Furthermore, cycle touring bikes are typically equipped differently from the simple bike setups used by locals. The brakes, gearing, handlebars, and saddles, as well as unfamiliarity with the types of locks or alarms in use, can pose a challenge. Consequently, when fully loaded, your bike is often of little interest to thieves. Your bags or other belongings are more valuable.

Although bicycles may not be a common target for theft in Southeast Asia, securing them with a lock is still advisable to prevent opportunistic theft. Thieves may wheel or carry away a bicycle and loot unsecured bags before abandoning the bike. In these countries, theft and attacks against tourists can result in severe punishment as they may negatively impact the economy. Therefore, it is not worth the risk for thieves to steal from tourists. However, leaving your cycle unlocked and unattended may invite trouble regardless of the country you are in, so it's crucial to secure your belongings as best you can using any available means.

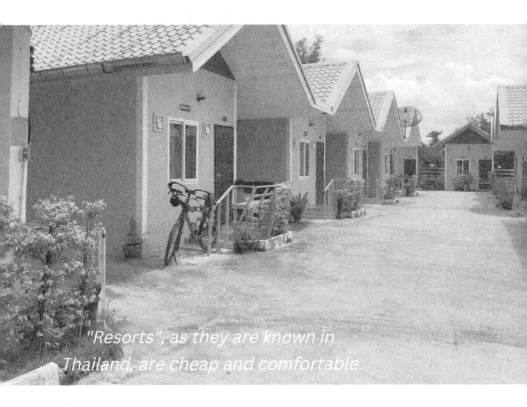
"Resorts", as they are known in Thailand, are cheap and comfortable.

One significant advantage of touring Southeast Asia is the abundance of affordable accommodation options such as hotels, guesthouses, and other lodging facilities. Self-contained, air-conditioned rooms are available at low prices, often cheaper than camping fees in Western countries. It's rare for a cyclist not to find a place to stay for the night within a day's ride. Moreover, bringing your gear inside the room or unit is typically hassle-free and accepted.

In Southeast Asia, most people attach little significance to your bike, and hotel management at more significant properties may request that you leave it outside or in the parking lot. Although this may frustrate cyclists who regard their bikes as a source of pride, hotel management views them as potential oil-dripping mud machines that could damage their flooring. From their perspective, it's understandable since most of us would want to avoid wheeling our cycles through our living rooms after a day's ride.

If possible, clean your bike before arriving at the hotel, especially if it looks muddy or dirty. A cleaner bike is more likely to be allowed in your room. In small resorts, your bike is more welcome. These inexpensive units typically include a bed, shower, air conditioning or fan, TV, Wi-Fi, and space to bring your bike inside for the night. These resorts are usually intended for short, temporary stays for drivers and other individuals working away from home. While they may not be the most luxurious places to stay, you can rest assured that your gear will be safe overnight.

Ensuring the safety of your bike during the day can be more challenging, which is why wheel locks, cables, and other mechanical devices are essential. When travelling with a partner or group, keeping your belongings safe becomes much easier. One person can enter a shop or establishment while the others keep an eye out. Some supermarkets may allow you to bring your bike inside, where you can leave it near the entrance or guards.

Physical harm is unlikely. As previously mentioned, there are severe punishments for those who harm tourists, so local thieves target locals instead. While being attacked is not common, it is not unheard of, so taking precautions is wise.

Nevertheless, it's always better to err on the side of caution. Therefore, wandering alone in unlit backstreets or similar areas late at night is not advisable. Even if you're looking for a shortcut back to your room, it's best to stick to well-lit and busy streets rather than back alleys.

It is essential to let someone know your whereabouts throughout the day. You can send a message to your family or friends, create a post on your social media if you use it, or inform the hotel or campsite staff about your expected return time if you plan to explore the town for entertainment or sightseeing. However, many Western travellers tend to feel much safer in Southeast Asia.

While some may feel anxious about travelling to certain parts of Southeast Asia, the region has a good safety reputation with little cause for concern.

It is crucial to avoid displaying valuable items while travelling, as motorcycle thieves are increasingly common. They can quickly snatch your mobile phone or bag while passing by, especially on busy streets filled with motorbikes and scooters, as is the case in Vietnam. So, it's best to handle your belongings discreetly and avoid doing so while in traffic. Again, this is a matter of common sense - things we wouldn't do in our own countries should also be avoided when travelling abroad.

If someone appears aggressive towards you, it's best to move away, but keep an eye on the person while doing so and not look away completely until you're out of harm's way. Although theft and violence can occur in any country, the likelihood of these happening to bicycle tourists in Southeast Asia is low based on statistics.

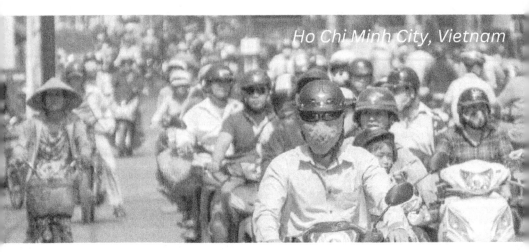
Ho Chi Minh City, Vietnam

Safety & Security

Thailand

Online tourism advice suggests that Thailand is a safe destination for tourists. However, visitors are advised to remain vigilant of potential dangers and security concerns that may arise.

Scams and fraud: Visitors need to be cautious about common scams prevalent in Thailand, such as overpriced goods or services, counterfeit or substandard products, and fraudulent money exchange schemes.

Petty crime: Pickpocketing, theft, and other petty crimes are common in high-traffic tourist areas. Visitors should exercise caution and be mindful.

Traffic safety: Traffic in Thailand can be chaotic, so road accidents are common. Visitors are advised to take precautions, such as helmets.

Natural disasters: Thailand is susceptible to natural disasters like floods and typhoons, so it's important to monitor local weather conditions and follow the advice of local authorities.

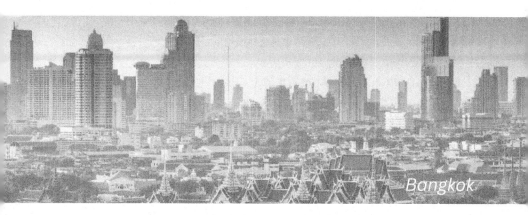
Bangkok

Political demonstrations: Thailand is prone to political demonstrations and rallies, which can cause travel disruptions and safety concerns. Although they are usually nonviolent, visitors should stay informed about the local political climate and avoid large gatherings.

Overall: Tourists can ensure their safety by exercising common sense and being mindful of their surroundings.

Laos

Online tourism advice: Laos is generally considered a safe destination for tourists. However, visitors should remain mindful of potential risks and inherent dangers when visiting a foreign country.

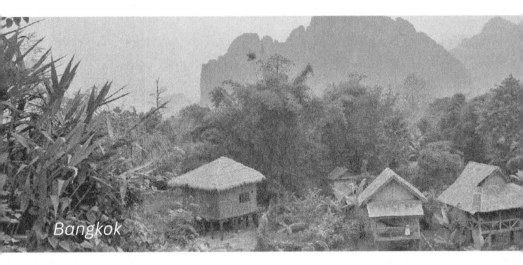

Bangkok

Road Safety: Road conditions can often be challenging, and accidents involving tourists have been reported. It's essential to exercise caution.

Scams: Like any tourist destination, Laos has its fair share of scams targeting travellers. Be cautious of individuals offering unofficial sightseeing or transport services at discounted prices, sometimes overpriced or unsafe.

Health Risks: Visitors to some areas of Laos should know that malaria and dengue fever are prevalent. Taking precautions, such as using insect repellent and taking the appropriate medications, is essential.

Political Instability: Although Laos is generally considered stable, incidents of political unrest have occurred in the past. Visitors should stay informed about the latest developments to ensure personal safety and avoid participating in large-scale demonstrations or rallies.

Overall: Exercise caution and remain aware of your surroundings. So tourists can have a safe and enjoyable trip to Laos.

Cambodia

Online tourism advice: Tourists in Cambodia face several potential dangers and security risks.

Pickpocketing and theft: Tourists should be cautious in Cambodia, especially in tourist areas and crowded public places.

Traffic accidents: The traffic in Cambodia can be chaotic and, at times, dangerous, and the roads are often poorly maintained.

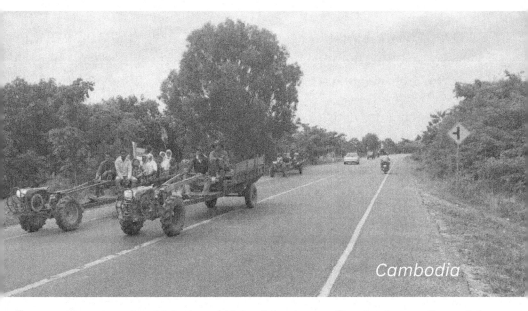

Cambodia

Scams: Tourists should be mindful of scams in Cambodia, such as fake police officers, overpriced goods and services, and fraudulent charities.

Health risks: Visitors should take necessary precautions to prevent food and water-borne illnesses and consider obtaining appropriate vaccinations.

Political instability: Political demonstrations in Cambodia can occur and, on occasion, turn violent, particularly in Phnom Penh.

Overall: Tourists in Cambodia should take necessary precautions, such as keeping valuables secure, following safe travel practices, and remaining aware of their surroundings.

Vietnam

Like any other country, Vietnam poses potential dangers and security concerns for tourists. However, with proper caution and awareness, most visitors can have a safe and enjoyable experience.

Crime: Pickpocketing and bag snatching are common occurrences in tourist areas in Vietnam. Visitors should be mindful of their belongings and avoid carrying valuables to prevent such incidents. Motorcycle thieves are also prevalent and may snatch valuables while passing by.

Scams: In Vietnam, some tourists have fallen victim to overcharging or scams by taxi drivers, street vendors, and tour operators. To avoid such issues, research common scams and negotiate prices beforehand.

Traffic: Vietnam has a high rate of road accidents due to heavy traffic and an increased number of motorbikes. So visitors should exercise extra caution when cycling.

Health: When travelling in Vietnam, there are health risks, such as food and water-borne illnesses and mosquito-borne diseases like dengue fever and malaria. To reduce the risk of such illnesses, visitors should take proper precautions, such as drinking bottled water and using insect repellent.

Political instability: Although Vietnam is stable, there are reports of politically motivated incidents of violence. Visitors should avoid political gatherings and demonstrations and monitor local news and travel alerts.

Overall: By taking the necessary precautions, such as being aware of surroundings and valuables, researching an area you plan to visit, and understanding local laws and customs, visitors can ensure a safe and enjoyable trip to Vietnam.

NOTES

DRAWING

CHAPTER SIX
Food & Phrases

Southeast Asian cuisine is renowned for its unique flavours, combining salty, sweet, sour, and spicy tastes. Food is often a top reason why cycle tourists return to Southeast Asia since cycle touring is about more than just pedalling. The cuisine uses lemongrass, fish sauce, chilli peppers, coconut milk, and lime. It is usually served with rice and is known for its balance of textures, including a mix of crunchy, chewy, and tender elements. Many dishes have been influenced by neighbouring countries like China and India, adding to the diversity of the cuisine.

Improving nutrition is a top priority for many regional governments in Southeast Asia due to high malnutrition and undernutrition rates, particularly in children. The growing burden of non-communicable diseases is also related to poor diet and nutrition. However, agricultural and food systems face challenges in producing and delivering nutritious food to all populations while promoting economic growth and development. Therefore, promoting good health and reducing poverty through improved nutrition is crucial for driving economic growth in Southeast Asia.

We aim to provide a simple guide to popular foods in each region you may visit on your ride. We have included translations in both English and local languages so that you can better communicate your food preferences to restaurant owners, cafes, and roadside shops.

Nothing is more frustrating than struggling to convey what you want, especially if locals do not understand your language or gestures due to cultural differences or misconceptions about tourists.

Thailand

Thai cuisine is renowned for balancing sweet, sour, salty, and spicy flavours with fresh herbs and spices. Street food vendors and markets are prevalent, offering traditional and fusion meals. Thai cuisine also uses dipping sauces like sweet chilli sauce, peanut sauce, and nam pla (fish sauce). Thai food is a mouth-watering combination of flavours and textures, utilising fresh ingredients to produce flavorful and satisfying dishes. So whether you're in the mood for a spicy soup, a sweet dessert, or a savoury stir-fry, Thai cuisine has something to offer every hungry cyclist.

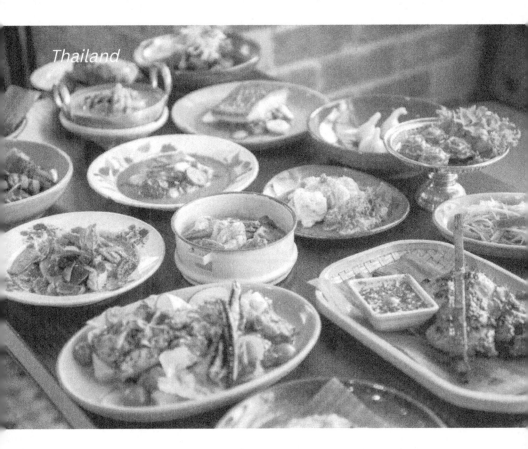

Thailand

Cycling along or near coastlines or at high altitudes, like mountains and hilly areas, can provide cooler air, making it more comfortable for cyclists. Conversely, lower areas and forested or jungle regions can have higher heat and humidity, making cycling more challenging.

A lousy stomach can be a nightmare for cycle tourists. Certain Thai foods may cause digestive discomfort for some individuals, while others may not be affected. For example, spicy dishes may contain chilli peppers, such as tom yum soup and green curry; raw or undercooked seafood dishes, like som tum (papaya salad), and fried foods, such as pad Thai or spring rolls, can trigger stomach issues. Foods with high levels of sugar or MSG, such as sweet and sour sauce or processed meat, can also cause discomfort. Additionally, street food or vendors may sometimes not adhere to hygiene standards, so it's essential to be cautious, mainly if your digestive system is not accustomed to the local cuisine.

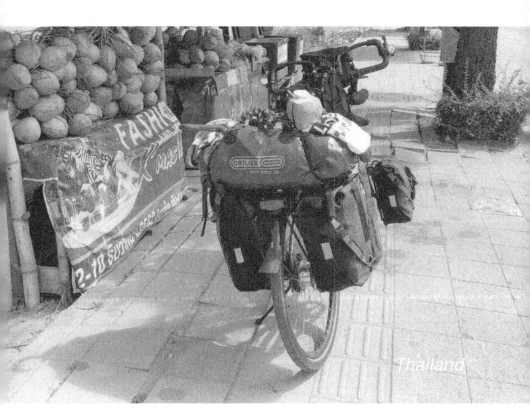

Thailand

Popular Dishes

- Mango Sticky Rice - ข้าวเหนียวมะม่วง - pronounced: "Khawhheniyw maṁwng" is sweet sticky rice served with sliced mango and topped with coconut milk.
- Fried Rice - ข้าวผัด - pronounced: "Khaw phad" is a simple dish of stir-fried rice with vegetables and your choice of protein.
- Roti - รกี - pronounced: "Rthi" is a simple batter fried on a hotplate with eggs and sugar and drizzled with condensed milk.
- Khao Soi - ข้าวซอย - pronounced: "Khawsxy" is a Northern Thai dish of egg noodles in a rich, creamy curry sauce with pickled mustard greens and crispy noodles on top.
- Som tum - ส้มตำ - pronounced: "Smta" is a spicy green papaya salad.
- Tom Yum Soup - ต้มยำ -pronounced: "Tmya" is a hot and sour soup with lemongrass, kaffir lime leaves, and chilli paste.
- Green Curry - แกงเขียวหวาน - pronounced: "Kaeng kheiywhwan" is a spicy curry made with coconut milk, green chilli, and various vegetables.
- Pad Thai - ผัดไทย - pronounced: "Phad thiy" is a stir-fried noodle with vegetables, peanuts, and your choice of protein.
- Kaeng Matsaman - แกงมัสมั่น - pronounced: "Kaeng masman" is a mild curry made with potatoes, peanuts and a choice of protein.
- Papaya Salad - ส้มตำปู - pronounced: "Smta pu" is a spicy salad made with shredded green papaya, tomatoes, peanuts, and dried shrimp.
- Pad Krapow - ผัดกะเพรา - pronounced: "Phad kaphera" consists of stir-fried pork, holy basil, garlic, fish sauce, and chilli peppers. It is usually served with jasmine rice and a fried egg on top.
- Drunken Noodles - ผัดขี้เมา - pronounced: "Phad khi mea" is stir-fried noodles with holy basil and lots of chillies. It's a cult-favourite Thai street food.
- Tom Kha Gai - ต้มข่าไก่ - pronounced: "Tmkha ki" is a mild coconut and chicken soup with lemongrass, galangal, and makrut lime.
- Khao Pad Sapparod - ข้าวผัดสัปปะรด -pronounced: "Khaw phad sappa rd" is a famous fried rice with pineapple and shrimps. Curry powder, shrimp sauce, oyster sauce, and fish sauce.

Pronunciations are not easy, so showing a person the items in Thai is an option.

Food & Phrases

Everyday Foods

Basic Foods	Thai	Pronounce
1. Bread	1. ขนมปัง	1. Khnmpang
2. Eggs	2. ไข่	2. Khi
3. Milk	3. น้ำนม	3. Nm
4. Cheese	4. ชีส	4. Chis
5. Yoghurt	5. โยเกิร์ต	5. Yo keirt
6. Rice	6. ข้าว	6. Khaw
7. Pasta	7. พาสต้า	7. Phas ta
8. Meat	8. เนื้อ	8. Neux
9. Fish	9. ปลา	9. Pla
10. Vegetables	10. ผัก	10. Phak
11. Fruits	11. ผลไม้	11. Phl mi
12. Juice	12. น้ำผลไม้	12. Na phl mi
13. Water	13. น้ำ	13. Na
14. Tea	14. ชา	14. Cha
15. Coffee	15. กาแฟ	15. Kafae
16. Beer	16. เบียร์	16. Beiyr
17. Wine	17. ไวน์	17. Win
18. Soft drinks	18. น้ำอัดลม	18. Naxadlm
19. Butter	19. เนย	19. Ney
20. Olive oil	20. น้ำมันมะกอก	20. Naman makxk
21. Peanut butter	21. เนยถั่ว	21. Ney thaw
22. Jam	22. แยม / เจลลี่	22. Yaem
23. Honey	23. น้ำผึ้ง	23. Naphung
24. Ketchup	24. ซอสมะเขือเทศ	24. Sxs makheuxthes
25. Mayonnaise	25. มายองเนส	25. Ma yxng nes
26. Soy sauce	26. ซีอิ๊ว	26. Sixiw
27. Salt	27. เกลือ	27. Kelux
28. Sugar	28. น้ำตาล	28. Natal
29. Flour	29. แป้ง	29. Paeg
30. Rice flour	30. แป้งข้าวจ้าว	30. Paeg khaw caw
31. Tofu	31. เต้าหู้	31. Teahu
32. Nuts	32. ถั่ว	32. Thaw
33. Dried fruit	33. ผลไม้แห้ง	33. Phl mi haeng
34. Porridge Oats	34. ข้าวโอ๊ตโจ๊ก	34. Khaw xot cok

Pronunciations are not easy, so showing a person the items in Thai is an option.

Everyday Numbers and Phrases

Numbers and Phrases	Thai	Pronounce
1. One	1. หนึ่ง	1. Hnung
2. Two	2. สอง	2. Song
3. Three	3. สาม	3. Sam
4. Four	4. สี่	4. Si
5. Five	5. ห้า	5. Ha
6. Six	6. หก	6. Hok
7. Seven	7. เจ็ด	7. Chet
8. Eight	8. แปด	8. Paet
9. Nine	9. เก้า	9. Kao
10. Ten	10. สิบ	10. Sib
11. Stop	11. หยุด	11. Hyud
12. How much	12. เท่าไร	12. Theari
13. Very expensive	13. แพงมาก	13. Phaeng mak
14. Reduce the price	14. ลดราคา	14. Ld rakha
15. Restaurant	15. ร้านอาหาร	15. Ran xahar
16. Cafe	16. คาเฟ่	16. Khafe
17. Toilet/Bathroom	17. ห้องน้ำ	17. Hxngna
18. Hungry	18. หิว	18. Hiw
19. May I have the menu	19. ขอเมนูค่ะ	19. Khx menu kha
20. Vegetarian	20. มังสวิรัติ	20. Mangswirati
21. No sugar	21. ไม่มีน้ำตาล	21. Mimi natal
22. One more please	22. ขออีกหนึ่ง	22. Khx xik hnung
23. It hurts	23. มันเจ็บ	23. Man Ceb
24. Hospital	24. โรงพยาบาล	24. Rong phyabal
25. Call ambulance	25. เรียกรถพยาบาล	25. Reiyk rth phyabal
26. I am lost	26. ฉันหลงทาง	26. Chan hlng thang
27. Can you help	27. คุณช่วยได้ไหม	27. Khun chwy di him
28. Cheers	28. ไชโย	28. Chiyo
29. Male hello/goodbye	29. สวัสดีคร๊าบ	29. Swasdi krap
30. Female hello/goodbye	30. สวัสดีคะ	30. Swasdi kha
31. No	31. ไม่	31. Mi
32. Yes	32. ใช่	32. Chi
33. Bicycle shop	33. ร้านจักรยาน	33. Ran cakryan
34. Hotel	34. โรงแรม	34. Rongraem
35. Guesthouse	35. บ้านพัก	35. Banphak

Pronunciations are not easy, so showing a person the items in Thai is an option.

Laos

Laotian cuisine is renowned for its use of fresh herbs and spices, which impart a distinctive flavour to the food. Sticky rice, papaya salad, and larb (a meat salad) are among the most popular dishes in Laos. Traditional ingredients like lemongrass, kaffir lime leaves, and galangal root are also commonly used to enhance the dishes' taste. Additionally, Laos's cuisine has been heavily influenced by its neighbours, Thailand and Vietnam, resulting in a fusion of flavours and techniques.

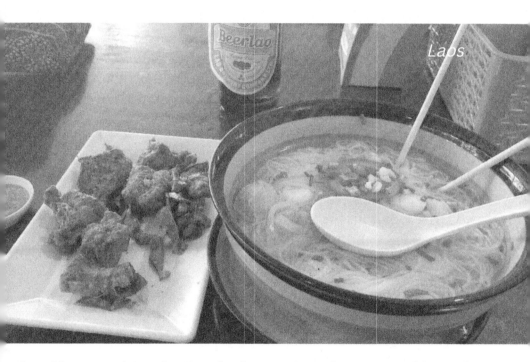

As with any cuisine, Laotian food can cause digestive problems if not handled, prepared, or stored correctly. For instance, eating undercooked or raw meats, consuming food left out at room temperature for extended periods, or drinking contaminated water can increase the chances of food poisoning. Furthermore, some individuals may have an intolerance or allergy to ingredients prevalent in Laos cuisine, such as peanuts or gluten. To minimise the likelihood of stomach upset, pay attention to your body and avoid consuming foods that have caused discomfort in the past.

Popular Dishes

- Papaya Salad - ຕໍາໝາກຫຸ່ງ - pronounced: "Tahm mahk hoong" is a cold salad with green papaya, garlic, spicy red chilli, fish sauce, shrimp paste, long bean, tomatoes, carrots and lime juice.
- Laap - ລາບ - pronounced: "Lahp" is minced meat and herb salad perfect for chicken, beef, tofu or veggies. Bursting with flavours of herbs and spices.
- Or Lam - ເອາະຫຼາມ - pronounced: "Oar lahm" is a mildly spicy, slightly tongue-numbing, Laotian stew.
- Jeow - ແຈວສົ້ມ - pronounced: "Jew" is a Laotian spicy and sour multiple-purpose dipping sauce. It can be used for meat, chicken, seafood, and veggies.
- Khao Piak Sen - ເຂົ້າເປຶຽກເສັ້ນ - pronounced: "Khow piak sen" is a traditional Lao noodle made of broth stewed with chicken, lemongrass, kaffir lime leaves, galangal, ginger, and soy sauce.
- Khao Jee - ເຂົ້າຈີ່ - pronounced: "Khow jee" is made when sticky rice is skewered and grilled with a brushing of egg to create a crispness.
- Nam Khao Tod - ໝ້ຳເຂົ້າຕົ້ມ - pronounced: "Nahm khow tohd" is made with jasmine rice balls coated in curry and herbs then deep fried; the fried rice balls are broken and mixed with fish sauce.
- Mok Pa - ໝົກປາ - pronounced: "Mok pah" is a famous steamed fish parcel from Laos made from white fish, herbs and seasonings, along with whole sticky rice grains.
- Kaipen - ໄຄແຜ່ນ - pronounced: "Kai-pen" is a Laotian snack made of freshwater green algae, garlic, vegetables, and sesame seeds.
- Ping Kai - ປຶ້ງໄກ່ - pronounced: "Ping kai" is the Lao version of grilled chicken. In Thailand it's also called kai yang, gai yang, kai ping, gai ping, or kai yang lao.
- Pho - ໂພ - pronounced: "Fuh." Vietnamese pho generally uses chicken or beef in the soup broth, whereas Lao pho often uses pork broth topped with crispy pork on top. The rice sticks used in Lao pho bowls are often thinner than Vietnamese.
- Khao Poon - ເຂົ້າປຸ້ນ - pronounced: "Khao pun" is often described as Lao royal vermicelli coconut curry soup due to its bright red and golden colors representing the colors of the Lao royal family.

Pronunciations are not easy, so showing a person the items in Laotian is an option.

Food & Phrases
Everyday Foods

Basic Foods	Laotian	Pronounce
1. Bread	1. ເຂົ້າຈີ່	1. Khao chi
2. Eggs	2. ໄຂ່	2. Khai
3. Milk	3. ນົມ	3. Nom
4. Cheese	4. ເນີຍແຂງ	4. Noeny aekhng
5. Yoghurt	5. ໂຍເກິດ	5. Oy koed
6. Rice	6. ເຂົ້າ	6. Khao
7. Pasta	7. Pasta	7. Pasta
8. Meat	8. ຊີ້ນ	8. Sin
9. Fish	9. ປາ	9. Pa
10. Vegetables	10. ຜັກ	10. Phak
11. Fruits	11. ໝາກໄມ້	11. Makmai
12. Fruit Juice	12. ນ້ຳໝາກໄມ້	12. Noa makmai
13. Water	13. ນ້ຳ	13. Noa
14. Tea	14. ຊາ	14. Sa
15. Coffee	15. ກາເຟ	15. Ka fe
16. Beer	16. ເບຍ	16. Bia
17. Wine	17. ເຫົ້າແວງ	17. Heoa aeuang
18. Soft drinks	18. ນ້ຳອັດລົມ	18. Noa ad lom
19. Butter	19. ມັນເບີ	19. Man boe
20. Olive oil	20. ນ້ຳມັນໝາກກອກ	20. N o a man mak kok
21. Peanut butter	21. ເນີຍຖົ່ວ	21. Noeny thov
22. Jam	22. Jam	22. Jam
23. Honey	23. ກຽດ	23. Kiad
24. Ketchup	24. Ketchup	24. Ketchup
25. Mayonnaise	25. ມາຍອນ	25. Ma yon
26. Soy sauce	26. ຊີ້ອີ້ວ	26. Su iv
27. Salt	27. ເກືອ	27. Keu
28. Sugar	28. ນ້ຳຕານ	28. Oatan
29. Flour	29. ແປ້ງ	29. Aepng
30. Rice flour	30. ແປ້ງເຂົ້າ	30. Aepng khao
31. Tofu	31. ເຕົ້າຫູ້	31. Tao hu
32. Nuts	32. ແກ່ນ	32. Aekn
33. Dried fruit	33. ໝາກໄມ້ແຫ້ງ	33. Makmai aehng
34. Porridge Oats	34. ເຂົ້າໂອດ	34. Khao ood

Pronunciations are not easy, so showing a person the items in Laotian is an option.

Everyday Numbers and Phrases

Numbers and Phrases	Laotian	Pronounce
1. One	1. ໜຶ່ງ	1. Nung
2. Two	2. ສອງ	2. Song
3. Three	3. ສາມ	3. Sam
4. Four	4. ສີ່	4. Si
5. Five	5. ຫ້າ	5. Ha
6. Six	6. ຫົກ	6. Hok
7. Seven	7. ເຈັດ	7. Ched
8. Eight	8. ແປດ	8. Aepd
9. Nine	9. ເກົ້າ	9. Kao
10. Ten	10. ສິບ	10. Sib
11. Stop	11. ຢຸດ	11. Yud
12. How much	12. ເທົ່າໃດ	12. Theoa dai
13. Very expensive	13. ແພງຫຼາຍ	13. Aephng rai
14. Reduce the price	14. ຫຼຸດລາຄາ	14. Rud lakha
15. Restaurant	15. ຮ້ານອາຫານ	15. Hanoahan
16. Cafe	16. ຮ້ານ	16. Han
17. Toilet/Bathroom	17. ຫ້ອງນ້ຳ	17. Hong nam
18. Hungry	18. ຫິວ	18. Hiv
19. May I have the menu	19. ຂ້ອຍຂໍເມນູ	19. Khonykho menu
20. Vegetarian	20. Vegetarian	20. Vegetarian
21. No sugar	21. ບໍ່ມີນ້ຳຕານ	21. Mimi natal
22. One more please	22. ກະລຸນາອີກອັນໜຶ່ງ	22. Kaluna ik annung
23. It hurts	23. ມັນເຈັບ	23. Man cheb
24. Hospital	24. ໂຮງໝໍ	24. Ohngmo
25. Call ambulance	25. ໂທຫາລົດສຸກເສີນ	25. Othha lod suksoen
26. I am lost	26. ຂ້ອຍເສຍ	26. Khony sia
27. Can you help	27. ເຈົ້າສາມາດຊ່ວຍໄດ້	27. Chao samadsuany dai
28. Cheers	28. ຊຸ່ມເຊຍ	28. Somsoeny
29. Hello	29. ສະບາຍດີ	29. Sabaidi
30. No	30. ບໍ່	30. Bo
31. Yes	31. ແມ່ນແລ້ວ	31. Aemnaelv
32. Bicycle shop	32. ຮ້ານຂາຍລົດຖີບ	32. Hankhai lodthib
33. Hotel	33. ໂຮງແຮມ	33. Ohngaehm
34. Guesthouse	34. ເຮືອນພັກ	34. Heuon phak

Pronunciations are not easy, so showing a person the items in Laotian is an option.

Cambodia

Cambodian cuisine is renowned for its distinctive flavour combinations, which blend sweet, sour, salty, and bitter tastes into the dishes. Popular ingredients include lemongrass, kaffir lime leaves, fish sauce, and prahok (fermented fish paste). Additionally, Cambodian cuisine typically employs a variety of fresh herbs, such as mint, cilantro, and basil, and is commonly served with rice. Some well-known dishes include amok (steamed fish in coconut curry), nom banh chok (rice noodles with a spicy fish-based sauce), and bai sach chrouk (pork and rice).

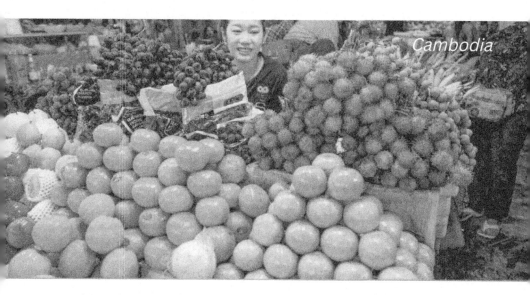
Cambodia

To avoid experiencing stomach upset when eating Cambodian food, it's advisable to follow these guidelines: drink only bottled water and avoid tap water, ice, and drinks prepared with tap water. Choose street food vendors with high turnover who maintain good hygiene practices. Ensure that food, especially meats, eggs, and seafood, is cooked thoroughly. Exercise caution when trying new foods, and begin with small portions to assess your body's response. Refrain from consuming raw or undercooked fruits and vegetables, particularly if rinsed in tap water. Wash your hands frequently and use hand sanitiser when hand-washing facilities are unavailable.

- Amok - អាម៉ុក - pronounced: "A mo k" in short, amok is a way of steam cooking a curry-flavoured protein like fish, beef, or chicken in a banana leaf.
- Bok L'hong - បុកល្ហុង - pronounced: "Bokalhoung" is the Cambodian version of green papaya salad that is prepared with crab, tomatoes, yardlong beans and peanuts.
- Kdam Chaa - ក្ដាមចៀន - pronounced: "Ktam cha nh" is Cambodia's favourite way of eating crab. Crabs are stir-fried with various ingredients, including green pepper from Kampot, Cambodia.
- Nom Banh Chok - នំបញ្ចុក - pronounced: "Nom ba nh chouk" are noodles laboriously crushed with rice, topped with lemongrass, rhizome, turmeric root, and other Cambodian ingredients.
- Khmer Red Curry - ខ្មែរការីវ៉ាស្ទី - pronounced "Khmer kari rea sai" is coconut-milk-based, made from beef, chicken or fish, eggplant, green beans, potatoes, fresh coconut milk, and lemongrass.
- Lap Khmer - ឡាបខ្មែរ - pronounced "La b khmer" is a minced beef salad with herbs and raw vegetables that is typical of Cambodian cuisine.
- Kuy Teav - គុយទាវ - pronounced: "Kouyteav" is made with beef stock, thinly sliced beef stock, garlic, onion, celery leaves, and noodles.
- Cha Houy Teuk - ចាហួយតឹក - pronounced: "Chahuoy toek" is a sweet jelly dessert – one of the most famous street foods in Cambodia.
- Bai Sach Chrouk - បៃសាច់ជ្រូង - pronounced: "Bai sach chhrao ng" is pork with rice and is one of Cambodia's most popular breakfasts.
- Char Kroeung Sach Ko - ចារគ្រឿងសាច់កោ - pronounced: "Char kroe ng sach kao" is a salty, sweet, and slightly spicy, stir-fried lemongrass with beef.
- Num Pang - នំបាង - pronounced: Nom Bang is a famous Cambodian sandwich with toasted baguette, pulled pork or other meat, pickled carrots or daikon, cilantro, chilli sauce, and pickles.
- Krolan - ក្រឡាញ - pronounced: "Kralea nh" is a rice pudding cooked in bamboo, sometimes with beans added.
- Chive Cakes - កាត់ពាក្ត - pronounced: "Keat pea k" are pan-fried snacks made with glutinous rice flour and chopped chives.

Pronunciations are not easy, so showing a person the items in Khmer is an option.

Food & Phrases
Everyday Foods

Basic Foods	Khmer	Pronounce
1. Bread	1. នំប៉័ង	1. Nombong
2. Eggs	2. ស៊ុត	2. Saout
3. Milk	3. ទឹកដោះគោ	3. Tukdaohko
4. Cheese	4. ឈីស	4. Chhi s
5. Yoghurt	5. ទឹកដោះគោជូរ	5. Tukdaohko chour
6. Rice	6. អង្ករ	6. Angkor
7. Pasta	7. ប៉ាស្តា	7. Ba sta
8. Meat	8. សាច់	8. Sach
9. Fish	9. ត្រី	9. Trei
10. Vegetables	10. បន្លែ	10. Banle
11. Fruits	11. ផ្លែឈើ	11. Phlechheu
12. Fruit Juice	12. ទឹកផ្លែឈើ	12. Tuk phlechheu
13. Water	13. ទឹក។	13. Tuk
14. Tea	14. តែ	14. Te
15. Coffee	15. កាហ្វេ	15. Kahve
16. Beer	16. ស្រាបៀរ	16. Srabie r
17. Wine	17. ស្រា	17. Sra
18. Soft drinks	18. ភេសជ្ជៈ	18. Phesachch
19. Butter	19. ប៊ី	19. Bu
20. Olive oil	20. ប្រេងអូលីវ	20. Breng au liv
21. Peanut butter	21. ប៊ីសណ្តែកដី	21. Bu sa nte k dei
22. Jam	22. យៈសាពូនមី	22. Y sa poun mi
23. Honey	23. ទឹកឃ្មុំ	23. Tukakhmoum
24. Ketchup	24. Ketchup	24. Ketchup
25. Mayonnaise	25. Mayonnaise	25. Mayonnaise
26. Soy sauce	26. ទឹកស៊ីអ៊ីវ	26. Tuk saiaiv
27. Salt	27. អំបិល	27. Ambel
28. Sugar	28. ស្ករ	28. Skar
29. Flour	29. ម្សៅ	29. Msaow
30. Rice flour	30. ម្សៅអង្ករ	30. Msaow angkor
31. Tofu	31. តៅហ៊ូ	31. Tawhou
32. Nuts	32. គ្រាប់	32. Kreab
33. Dried fruit	33. ផ្លែឈើស្ងួត	33. Phlechheu sngout
34. Porridge Oats	34. បបរ oats	34. Babr oats

Pronunciations are not easy, so showing a person the items in Khmer is an option.

Cycling Southeast Asia
Everyday Numbers and Phrases

Numbers and Phrases	Khmer	Pronounce
1. One	1. មួយ។	1. Muoy
2. Two	2. ពីរ	2. Pir
3. Three	3. បី	3. Bei
4. Four	4. បួន	4. Buon
5. Five	5. រាំ	5. Bram
6. Six	6. ប្រាំមួយ។	6. Bramuoy
7. Seven	7. រាំពីរ	7. Brapir
8. Eight	8. ប្រាំបី	8. Brabei
9. Nine	9. រាំបួន	9. Brabuon
10. Ten	10. ដប់	10. Db
11. Stop	11. ឈប់	11. Chhb
12. How much	12. ប៉ុន្មាន	12. Bonman
13. Very expensive	13. ថ្លៃណាស់	13. Thlai nasa
14. Reduce the price	14. កាត់បន្ថយតម្លៃ	14. Katbanthoy tamlei
15. Restaurant	15. ភោជនីយដ្ឋាន	15. Phochniyodthan
16. Cafe	16. ហាងកាហ្វេ	16. Hang kahve
17. Toilet/Bathroom	17. បង្គន់	17. Bangkon
18. Hungry	18. ឃ្លាន	18. Khlean
19. Menu	19. ម៉ឺនុយ	19. Meunouy
20. Vegetarian	20. បួស	20. Buos
21. No sugar	21. គ្មានជាតិស្ករ	21. Kmean cheate skar
22. One more	22. មួយទៀត	22. Muoytiet
23. It hurts	23. វាឈឺ	23. Vea Chhu
24. Hospital	24. មន្ទីរពេទ្យ	24. Montirpet
25. Ambulance	25. រថយន្តសង្គ្រោះ	25. Rothayont sangkroh
26. I am lost	26. ញុំវង្វេង	26. Khnhom vongveng
27. Help	27. ជំនួយ	27. Chomnuoy
28. Cheers	28. រីករាយ	28. Rikreay
29. Hello	29. ជំរាបសួរ	29. Chomreabsour
30. No	30. ទេ	30. Te
31. Yes	31. បាទ	31. Bat
32. Bicycle shop	32. ហាងកង់	32. Hang kng
33. Hotel	33. សណ្ឋាគារ	33. Santhakar
34. Guesthouse	34. ផ្ទះសំណាក់	34. Phteahsaamnak

Pronunciations are not easy, so showing a person the items in Khmer is an option.

Vietnam

Vietnamese cuisine is renowned for its harmonious blend of unique flavours. The food is made using fresh herbs, vegetables, and a variety of spices and sauces. Many dishes are carefully balanced to achieve a mix of flavours, such as sweet, sour, and salty, making them delicious and healthy. The combination of ingredients and flavours varies from region to region, resulting in diverse dishes. Vietnamese cuisine also features healthy cooking methods, such as steaming or grilling, that help retain the nutrients in the ingredients. In summary, Vietnamese food is delicious and nutritious, making it a crowd-pleaser.

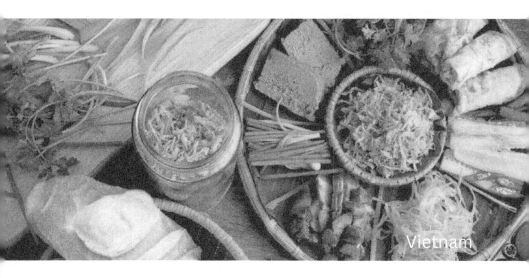

Vietnam

Stomach illnesses can be unpleasant, particularly when travelling to tropical climates like Vietnam. To minimize the risk of getting sick, it's advisable to follow these guidelines: drink only boiled or bottled water, wash your hands frequently with soap and water, and avoid raw fruits and vegetables unless you can peel them yourself. In addition, refrain from consuming street food unless thoroughly cooked and served hot. Avoid dairy products and ice as well. Finally, ensure that any fish or meat you consume is cooked through and served hot. While adhering to these recommendations is not always feasible, doing so can help reduce the risk of falling ill.

Popular Dishes

- Pho – Phở - pronounced: "Fuh" is a noodle soup made with beef, chicken, or seafood.
- Banh Mi - Bánh mì - pronounced: "Bun mee" is a sandwich made with a French baguette, pâté, mayonnaise, pickled vegetables, and fresh herbs.
- Bun Cha - Bún chả - pronounced: "Boon char" is a dish of grilled pork patties and pork belly served with vermicelli noodles.
- Goi Cuon - Gỏi cuốn - pronounced: "Goy kwon" is a fresh spring roll filled with pork, shrimp, and herbs.
- Com Tam - Cơm tấm - pronounced: "Gohm tam" is broken rice with grilled pork, fried egg, and other toppings.
- Cha Ca - Chả cá - pronounced: "Cha kah" made from fish paste mixed with rice flour, sometimes including dill, wrapped around bamboo sticks and grilled over charcoal.
- Banh Xeo - Bánh xèo - pronounced: "Bun say-oh" is a savoury crepe made with rice flour and filled with pork, shrimp, and bean sprouts
- Cao Lau - thick noodles served with pork, greens, and a special broth
- Bun Bo Hue - Bún bò Huế - pronounced: "Boon boh hway" is made with rice noodles, beef broth, and a variety of meats, including beef and pork, lemongrass, and chilli, with herbs and vegetables.
- Banh Cuon - Bánh cuốn - pronounced: "Bun kwon" is a steamed rice roll filled with pork and mushrooms.
- Xoi man - Xôi Mặn - pronounced: "Soy man" is sticky rice topped with pork, chicken, or vegetables.
- Banh Hoi - Bánh hỏi - pronounced: "Bun hoy" is made from thin rice vermicelli noodles woven into delicate bundles, grilled or steamed.
- Bot Loc - Bột lọc - pronounced: "Bawt lock" are tapioca dumplings filled with shrimp and pork.
- Ga Tan - Gà tần - pronounced: "Ga tawn" is a chicken soup with a combination of instant noodles, mugwort and oriental herbs.
- Bun Rieu - Bún Riêu - a noodle soup made with tomato and crab.
- Mi Quang - Mì Quảng - pronounced: "Mee quanhng" is thick noodles served with shrimp, pork, and a special broth.

Pronunciations are not easy, so showing a person the items in Vietnamese is an option.

Food & Phrases
Everyday Foods

Basic Foods	Vietnamese	Pronounce
1. Bread	1. Bánh mì	1. Bun mee
2. Eggs	2. Trứng	2. Tung
3. Milk	3. Sữa	3. Soo-ah
4. Cheese	4. Phô mai	4. Fuh my
5. Yoghurt	5. Sữa chua	5. Soo-ah choo-ah
6. Rice	6. Cơm	6. Gohm
7. Pasta	7. Mỳ ống	7. Mee yong
8. Meat	8. Thịt	8. Teet
9. Fish	9. Cá	9. Cah
10. Vegetables	10. Rau	10. Rau
11. Fruits	11. Trái cây	11. Trie chai
12. Fruit Juice	12. Nước trai cây	12. Noo-awk trie chai
13. Water	13. Nước	13. Nook
14. Tea	14. Trà	14. Tah
15. Coffee	15. Cà phê	15. Cah feh
16. Beer	16. Bia	16. Bee-ah
17. Wine	17. Rượu	17. Rwow
18. Soft drinks	18. Nước ngọt	18. Noo-awk noht
19. Butter	19. Bơ	19. Buh
20. Olive oil	20. Dầu ô liu	20. Dow oh lee-oo
21. Peanut butter	21. "Bơ đậu phộng	21. Buh dau fong
22. Jam	22. Mứt	22. Moot
23. Honey	23. Em yêu	23. Em yuh
24. Ketchup	24. Sốt cà chua	24. Sot cah choo-ah
25. Mayonnaise	25. Mayonaise	25. Mayonnaise
26. Soy sauce	26. Xì dầu	26. See dau
27. Salt	27. Muối	27. Moo-oy
28. Sugar	28. Đường	28. Dwong
29. Flour	29. Bột mì	29. Bawt mee
30. Rice flour	30. Bột gạo	30. Bawt gow
31. Tofu	31. Đậu hũ	31. Dau hoo
32. Nuts	32. Quả hạch	32. Kwah hahch
33. Dried fruit	33. Hoa quả sấy khô	33. Ho-ah kwah say kho
34. Porridge Oats	34. Cháo yến mạch	34. Chow yen mahch

Pronunciations are not easy, so showing a person the items in Vietnamese is an option.

Cycling Southeast Asia
Everyday Numbers and Phrases

Numbers and Phrases	Vietnamese	Pronounce
1. One	1. Một	1. Moot
2. Two	2. Hai	2. Hi
3. Three	3. Ba	3. Bah
4. Four	4. Bốn	4. Bawn
5. Five	5. Năm	5. Nohm
6. Six	6. Sáu	6. Sow
7. Seven	7. Bảy	7. By
8. Eight	8. Tám	8. Tahm
9. Nine	9. Chín	9. Cheen
10. Ten	10. Mười	10. Moo-oy
11. Stop	11. Dừng lại	11. Dung lai
12. How much	12. Bao nhiêu	12. Bao nyee-uh
13. Very expensive	13. Rất đắt	13. Rat daht
14. Reduce the price	14. Giảm giá	14. Jeem gia
15. Restaurant	15. Nhà hàng	15. Nah hang
16. Cafe	16. Quán cà phê	16. Kwan ca fey
17. Toilet/Bathroom	17. Phòng vệ sinh	17. Fong vay sinh
18. Hungry	18. Đói bụng	18. Doy bung
19. Menu	19. Thực đơn	19. Took dawn
20. Vegetarian	20. Người ăn chay	20. Ngoo-ey un chai
21. No sugar	21. Không đường	21. Khong dwong
22. One more	22. Một lần nữa	22. Moot lahn nuh-ah
23. It hurts	23. Nó đau	23. No daw
24. Hospital	24. Bệnh viện	24. Behn vyen
25. Call ambulance	25. Gọi xe cấp cứu	25. Go-ee say cap coo
26. I am lost	26. Tôi bị lạc	26. Toy bee lak
27. Can you help	27. Bạn có thể giúp	27. Bahn co tay joop
28. Cheers	28. Chúc mừng	28. Chook mung
29. Hello	29. Xin chào	29. Sin chow
30. No	30. KHÔNG	30. Kohng
31. Yes	31. Đúng	31. Dawng
32. Bicycle shop	32. Cửa hàng xe đạp	32. Koo-ah hang say dap
33. Hotel	33. Khách sạn	33. Khach san
34. Guesthouse	34. Nhà khách	34. Nah khach

Pronunciations are not easy, so showing a person the items in Vietnamese is an option.

DRAWING

CHAPTER SEVEN
Getting There

There are many good reasons why someone might bring a bike to Southeast Asia instead of relying on other forms of transportation upon arrival. For one, cycling offers a more immersive and adventurous way to experience Southeast Asia's local culture and scenery.

Cycling is a great way to stay active and maintain fitness while travelling. It is, quite often, a more cost-effective mode of transportation. Additionally, it is a sustainable and eco-friendly travel method, reducing carbon emissions. Cycling also provides greater flexibility and independence during your travels, enabling you to take detours, make unscheduled stops, and explore at your own pace. Offering the opportunity to interact with local communities and experience the culture uniquely and personally, creating lasting memories and a deeper connection to the places you visit.

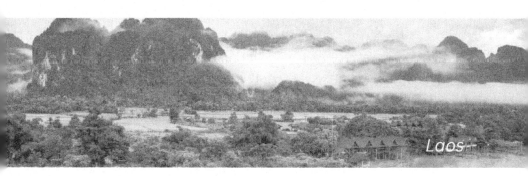

Laos

Travelling overland to Southeast Asia on long tours is popular for many cyclists. However, for most travellers, flying into a major city airport and departing from there is the most common method.

Transporting the bike and gear can be a major concern for many travellers, as some airlines may not make it easy. In some cases, the weight of the cycle and gear may be light enough to be covered by the baggage allowance. However, the combined weight of the bike and equipment, including clothing and other items, will often exceed the baggage allowance.

Transporting a bike as additional luggage can be relatively inexpensive or even free when travelling within a large country or to a neighbouring country, such as Europe or another state in countries like the United States. However, if you need to transport a bike halfway around the world, be prepared to pay a premium unless you find a great deal by chance.

Transporting a bike can sometimes cost more than the cyclist's seat price, which may seem excessive. However, it is worth it, especially if you travel with a bike that suits your needs and preferences. Ideally, it would be best to include the cycle in your baggage allowance and pack the gear as hand luggage in a rack-pack or a foldable hold all.

To ensure that your bike box is secure and to facilitate an inspection, it is best to seal and tape it thoroughly before cutting small holes near each tyre to serve as inspection ports and allow staff to verify that you have let the tyre pressure down if required. It might deter anyone from opening the box, damaging your bike, or improperly securing it afterwards.

There are different opinions on whether letting the tyre pressure down helps during air travel, but if your airline mandates it, it is advisable to comply. You do not need to release all the air, just enough to ensure that the tyres can accommodate changes in altitude and pressure during the flight.

If the combined weight of your bike and cardboard box is below the weight limit set by your airline, you may consider using the remaining allowance to pack some of your gear inside the box to provide extra cushioning for your bike. Items such as your sleeping bag, tent, clothing, or empty panniers can serve as padding and help protect your bike during transit. However, securing these items to the bike frame is essential if the box gets opened or damaged during handling.

It may seem unlikely that a tyre could burst under pressure during a flight, but it is still best to comply with the airline if they request it. Deflating does not take much time and can help prevent any potential issues.

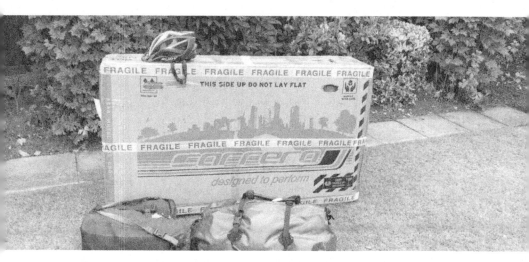

While some domestic flights in certain countries may allow you to bring your bike on the plane as it is, on most long-haul flights, where space in the cargo hold is limited, airlines typically require you to pack your bike in a specific box or bag of a certain size and weight.

Depending on the airline's requirements, you may need to disassemble your bike partially before packing it. This may involve removing the seat and seat post, pedals, handlebars, stem, forks, and front and rear wheels. Once disassembled, you can secure the wheels to the sides of the bike using cable ties or tape, avoiding brown box tape that can be difficult to remove and may damage the paint. For added protection, you can use fork spacers, disc brake protectors, and sprocket protectors, often free at bike shops.

Cardboard boxes are a great option for packing your bike, and you can quickly dispose of them at your destination by leaving them at the airport. Some cyclists even search for leftover boxes at airports. Cardboard provides excellent protection against scratches and dents and has the added benefit of being able to slide smoothly. Baggage handlers have reported that sliding baggage is easier to move and stack than plastic materials like shrink wrap or bubble wrap, which can stick to floors, truck beds, or ramps and cause handlers to throw the luggage instead.

Finding a suitable cardboard box for your bike is usually fine, as they are widely available in most towns worldwide. In many countries, bike shops or other businesses may provide them for free, while in some poorer countries, locals may ask for a small fee in exchange for a box.

Adherence to your chosen airline's guidelines when packing your bike is essential. If the airline specifies the box's maximum size and weight, it is best to comply. Also, if the airline requires you to deflate the bike's tires, it would be best to do so. While you may have personal reservations about these rules, arguing with the staff is not a good idea.

Some airlines may charge a high fee for transporting a bike, sometimes more significant than a person's airfare. If you find yourself in this situation, it is worth inquiring about paying for a seat upgrade. This could save you money while allowing you to bring your bike on the flight.

Suppose your seat costs US$700, and you have been quoted US$500 for the bike. Before paying, consider inquiring about any available upgrades, such as Premium or Business Class seats. These upgraded tickets usually offer a significantly larger baggage allowance, potentially covering your cycle or gear.

While the cost will remain US$1200, upgrading to a more luxurious option will ensure you travel comfortably, enjoy superior cuisine, and receive priority boarding. This will result in a more pleasant travel experience and leave you feeling rejuvenated upon arrival. Additionally, you might even feel energized enough to leave the airport and begin your journey straight away. Although it may cost the same amount, the added comfort and benefits make it a worthwhile investment.

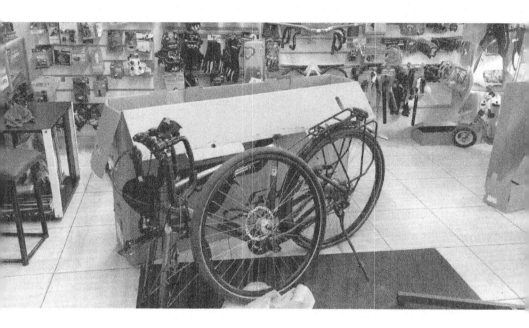

Whether you're embarking on a cycling tour or returning home or to another destination, it can be beneficial and cost-effective to drop off your cycle at a local bike shop to have it boxed if you're not comfortable dismantling it yourself. This option is handy, depending on your location. You may even be able to help the bike mechanic and learn how to reassemble your cycle at your destination. Although this service can be costly, bike shops can often provide boxes promptly and help you arrange local transportation to the airport for you when your flight is scheduled.

Not everyone has a secure location to store a plastic or metal bike case while away from home, making a cardboard bike box a practical option. Regardless of the packaging material, it's crucial to ensure that all individual bike components are securely fastened together to prevent any parts from getting lost in case the packaging is opened.

You can locate self-storage facilities, especially if you're flying to a location and embarking on a cycling tour before returning to the same airport for your flight home. In this case, you could opt for a more expensive, reusable bike storage case. Then, once you have rebuilt your cycle at your destination, you could drop off the storage case at a self-storage facility or rebuild the bike at the storage facility. Although the cost of storing such a small item shouldn't be high, having a secure case waiting for you is worth the peace of mind instead of searching for a cardboard bike box. However, if you're returning home from the same airport and the storage cost is low, you could also use a cardboard bike box. Also, you can find a contact at your destination ahead of time who can keep your box safe.

Depending on your location, it can often be helpful and cost-effective to drop off your cycle at a local bike shop for boxing before embarking on your cycling tour, returning home, or travelling to another destination. This option is handy for those who need more confidence in dismantling their bike. Often, individuals have the opportunity to assist the bike mechanic and gain an understanding of how to reassemble their cycle at their destination. In addition, this service is typically reasonably priced, and some shops can quickly obtain boxes and even arrange for local transportation to the airport when your flight is scheduled.

Dedicated Cycle Bag

Pros

1. Convenience: Bicycle bags are convenient for solo travellers as they are lighter and make it difficult for anyone to see what is inside.
2. Cost: Dedicated bags are usually less expensive hard-shell cases, making them more affordable for transporting your bike via air travel. However, cardboard boxes may be available at no cost.
3. Space-saving: Dedicated bags are designed to be compact and easy to store when not in use, making them an ideal choice for individuals with limited storage space. Additionally, they can be stored in a pannier for the return flight.

Cons

1. Protection: While bicycle bags can offer some protection during transport, they are generally less durable than bike boxes or hard-shell cases, increasing the risk of damage to your bike while travelling.
2. Regulations: It's important to note that different airlines have varying requirements for how cycles should be packed for air travel, and bicycle bags may need to meet these specific regulations. This could result in additional fees or restrictions on transporting your bike.
3. Assembly: Disassembling and reassembling your bike can take time, mainly if you are unfamiliar with the process. Furthermore, if parts of your bike are damaged during transport, it may not be easy to repair once you reach your destination.

Clear Plastic Cycle Bag

<u>Pros</u>

1. Cost: Clear plastic bags are usually more affordable than bike boxes, hard-shell cases, or dedicated bags, making them a budget-friendly choice for transporting your bike by air.
2. Lightweight: Clear plastic bags are lightweight and easy to handle, making them a convenient option for solo travellers.

<u>Cons</u>

1. Protection: Clear plastic bags do not provide substantial protection for your bike during transport and are not as durable as bike boxes or hard-shell cases, making them a high-risk option for damage during travel.
2. Regulations: Airlines have specific requirements for packing bicycles for air travel, and clear plastic bags may need to meet these requirements. This can result in additional fees or restrictions on transportation.
3. Visibility: Clear plastic bags make it easier for baggage handlers to see the contents of your bag, which can increase the risk of theft or damage to your bike during transport.
4. Assembly: Disassembling and reassembling your bike can be time-consuming, especially if you are unfamiliar with it. Additionally, if any parts of your bike are damaged during transport, it can be challenging to repair your bike once you arrive at your destination.

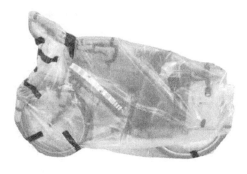

Cardboard Cycle Box

Pros

1. Protection: Compared to clear plastic bags, cardboard bike boxes offer more substantial protection for your bike during transport. This can help reduce the risk of damage during travel, and they can often be obtained for free or at a low cost.
2. Regulations: Many airlines have specific requirements for packing bicycles for air travel, and cardboard bike boxes are typically compliant. This can minimize the risk of additional fees or restrictions.
3. Durability: Cardboard bike boxes are sturdier than clear plastic bags, making them less likely to be damaged during transit.
4. Reusable: Unlike clear plastic bags, which are typically single-use, cardboard bike boxes are more environmentally friendly and can be reused.
5. It can often be got for little or no money.

Cons

1. Durability: While cardboard bike boxes are sturdier than clear plastic bags, they are still made of cardboard and can be easily damaged if not handled properly. Furthermore, they are not as durable as hard-shell cases, so there is still a risk of damage during transit.

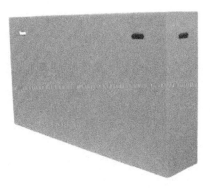

Cycle Box

<u>Pros</u>

1. Protection: Bicycle boxes offer high protection for your bike during transit, reducing the risk of damage during travel.
2. Regulations: Many airlines have specific requirements for packing bikes for travel, and bicycle boxes are often compliant with these requirements, which can minimize the risk of additional fees or restrictions on the transportation of your bike.
3. Durability: Bicycle boxes are made of sturdy materials like plastic or hardshell, making them less likely to be damaged during transit than cardboard boxes or clear plastic bags.
4. Reuse: Bicycle boxes can be reused multiple times, making them a more eco-friendly and cost-effective option for transporting your bike by air.

<u>Cons</u>

1. Cost: While bicycle boxes can provide excellent protection for your bike, they are typically more expensive than clear plastic bags or cardboard boxes. Additionally, finding a place to store the box for your return trip can take time and effort.
2. Assembly: Assembling and disassembling your bike from a compact bike box can take time, especially if you are still familiar with the process. However, some boxes are more spacious than others.
3. Weight: Bicycle boxes can be heavy and awkward to handle. Opting for a wheeled version is a good idea.
4. Size: Bicycle boxes can be bulky and oddly shaped, making them difficult to store when not in use.

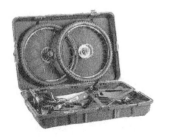

Getting There

Let's break down the various ways to get there with a bike:

Air Travel: You can bring your bicycle on a plane as checked baggage, but most airlines charge a fee for this service and have specific restrictions regarding the bike's size and weight.

Overland Travel: If you're starting from a nearby country, you can travel overland to Southeast Asia with your bicycle. This may entail taking trains, buses, or other modes of transportation and or simply cycling a border crossing.

Cycling: You can opt for a cycle tour, individually or with a group, taking you from one country to another. This type of travel is perfect for those who prefer an active and independent style of travel. But, again, you can search for plenty of options online.

Shipping: Another alternative is to ship your bicycle to Southeast Asia and collect it when you arrive. This can be a convenient option if you're flying and want to avoid the hassle of transporting your bicycle on the plane.

- While catching a ship to Southeast Asia can be challenging, it is still possible. However, the most common method of transporting a bicycle to Southeast Asia is by ship while you take a flight, but timing can take work.

- Disassemble your bike as much as you need to and place it in a durable box or bike bag to pack it correctly. Ensure to pad and protect components.

- Research shipping options. Look for companies that can provide bike shipping services to Southeast Asia. Compare prices, transit times, and available services to find the best option.

- Secure the necessary documentation, including commercial invoice, bill of lading, and other paperwork to clear customs, depending on the destination country.

- Once you have selected a shipping company and method, you can book the shipment and pay the necessary fees.

- Prepare the bike for pickup or delivery by ensuring it is packed and ready to go on the scheduled day.

- Track the shipment to monitor its progress and estimate its arrival time.

Note: Before shipping, check the regulations and customs requirements for importing bikes in the destination country. Also, remember that arrival dates and times can change due to weather and other circumstances.

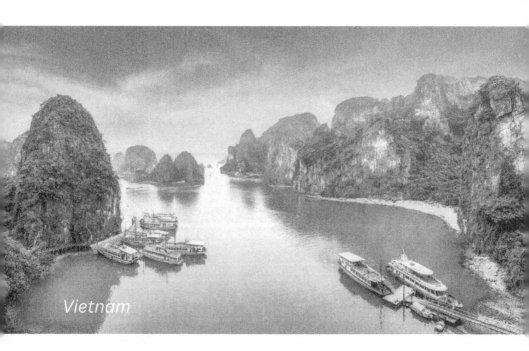

Vietnam

CHAPTER EIGHT
Places To Stay

In general, finding places to stay in Southeast Asia is relatively easy as many options are available, from budget-friendly hostels to luxury hotels. However, the ease of finding accommodation can vary depending on the location and time of year.

Popular tourist destinations like Kampot or Phuket offer many accommodation options, including hotels, resorts, and even Airbnb. In more rural areas, you may need to conduct more research to find a suitable place to stay, but it is usually a manageable challenge. It can sometimes be best to book accommodation in advance in certain areas during peak tourist season to secure the best options. However, most people can easily find places to stay on the day if they are open to unrated properties.

In addition to hotels and resorts, Southeast Asia also offers many homestays and guesthouses, which can provide a more authentic and immersive travel experience. For those seeking a more rugged or outdoor-oriented experience, many camping grounds and national parks in the region offer camping facilities.

In addition to hotels and resorts, Southeast Asia offers many homestays and guesthouses, which can provide a more authentic and immersive travel experience.

For those seeking a more rugged experience, many camping grounds and national parks in the region offer camping facilities. We will list just a few to give you an idea.

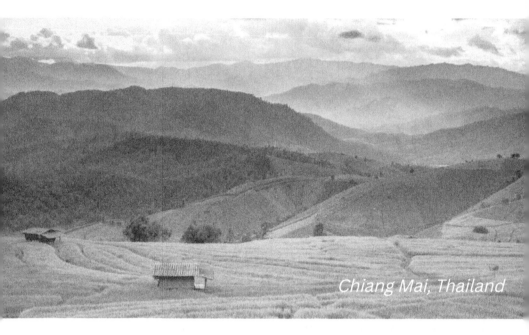

Chiang Mai, Thailand

Camping

Thailand

Camping in Thailand is an excellent way to experience the country's natural beauty and culture. Thailand boasts many stunning beaches, national parks, and other areas that offer camping opportunities.

When camping, being mindful of the local environment and wildlife is crucial. Protecting yourself from insect bites and other health risks is also essential. Following camping regulations and respecting the local culture and customs is important.

Whether you are a seasoned or a first-timer, camping in Thailand can be a unique and rewarding experience.

Some of Thailand's more popular tent campsites are in the south. However, there are many campsites throughout Thailand and plenty of places to stealth or wild camp. As with much of Southeast Asia, it is best to camp in established sites or well-trodden areas, as landmines and other unexploded ordinances are still risky.

A few of the many popular campsites

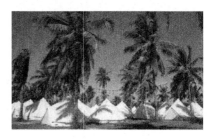

1 - Waterfront Camping
50 Moo 9 T Tambon Pong, Amphoe Bang Lamung, Chang Wat Chon Buri 20150

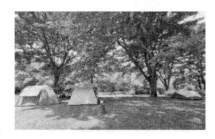

2 - Bambusa Camp
Tambon Klat Luang, Amphoe Tha Yang, Chang Wat Phetchaburi 76130

3 - Phu Chom Dao Campground
Bambusa Camp Tambon Klat Luang, R9MR+F5C, Wichit, Mueang Phuket District, Phuket 83000

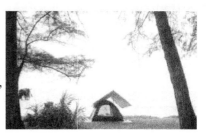

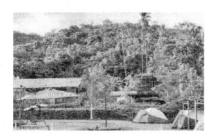

4 - Samui Camping Farm
122/45 Namuang, Ko Samui District, Surat Thani 84140

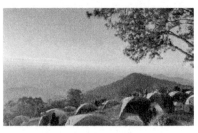

5 - Doi Pui Camping Area
Suthep, Mueang Chiang Mai District, Chiang Mai 50200

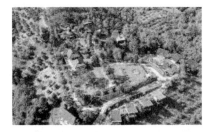

6 - Pilok Camp View
4088 Tambon Pilok, Amphoe Thong Pha Phum, Chang Wat Kanchanaburi 71180

7 - River Hill Camping
8, Tambon Thung Khwai Kin, Amphoe Klaeng, Chang Wat Rayong 21110

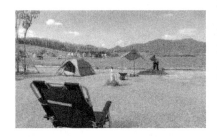

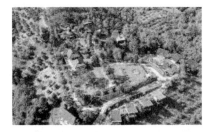

8 - Hilltop Retreat
Amphoe Lom Sak, Chang Wat Phetchabun 67110

9 - Uncle Charles's Camping
Tambon Khanong Phra, Amphoe Pak Chong, Chang Wat Nakhon Ratchasima 30130

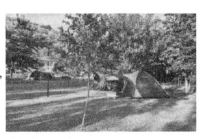

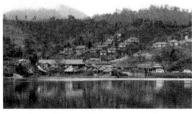

10 - Ban Rak Thai Lakefront Campsite
Ban Rak Thai, Tambon Mok Cham Pae, Amphoe Mueang Mae Hong Son, Chang Wat Mae Hong Son 58000

Laos

<u>Camping</u>

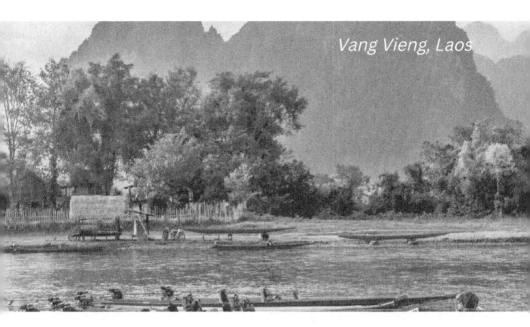

Vang Vieng, Laos

Camping in Laos is a popular activity for tourists who seek to experience the country's natural beauty, pristine landscapes, and cultural richness. Laos boasts several national parks and wilderness areas that are perfect for camping. Popular camping spots include Phou Khao Khouay National Park, Nam Ha National Protected Area, and the Bolaven Plateau.

Camping in Laos is generally safe, but taking precautions is essential to protect yourself from the elements, wildlife, and insects. Always carry a first-aid kit, plenty of water, and a map or GPS device. Letting someone know your plans and expected return time is also essential. Laos has a rich cultural heritage, and respecting local customs and traditions is crucial. Dress modestly and be mindful of local customs when interacting with people in rural areas. Overall, camping in Laos can be a wonderful experience for those who enjoy nature, outdoor adventure, and cultural immersion. You can enjoy a safe and unforgettable camping trip in this beautiful country with proper preparation and precautions.

To escape from the often oppressive heat and humidity of Southeast Asia, heading to the hills or coastlines is often the best option. The northern parts of these regions are hilly, but it is in the south where Cambodia has its highest hills.

Campsites are limited, but here are a few

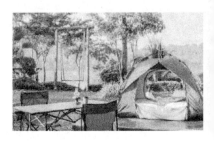

1 - River Moon Camping
Ban Ang

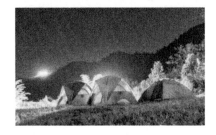

2 - Phoukhoun Backpacker and Camping
Phou Khoun

3 - Phachalern Camping Farm
See location 3 at the end of these regions'
campsite pages.

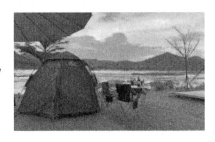

While there are several campsites visible on maps, there are undoubtedly many others that need to be marked. Additionally, plenty of resort-style guesthouses may allow tents to be pitched within their grounds. It is also worth noting that many temples throughout Southeast Asia are happy to accept guests free of charge. You may often find a place within the temple grounds or facilities to set up your tent or inner tent.

Cambodia

Camping

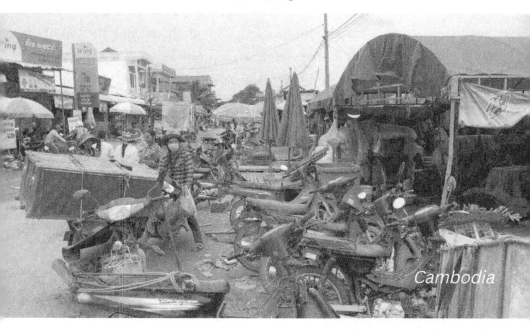

Cambodia

Camping in Cambodia can be an exciting experience, with diverse landscapes and natural attractions, such as towering hills, vast stretches of flat terrain, a scenic coastline, and bustling cities. However, be prepared for high temperatures during the day and cooler temperatures at night.

Cambodia boasts many stunning camping sites, including national parks and beaches, where you can pitch your tent and admire the breathtaking scenery. Some popular camping spots include Kirirom National Park, Bokor National Park, and Ream National Park.

Cambodia is generally safe for tourists, but it is always essential to take precautions, particularly when camping in remote areas. Make sure to research where you plan to camp and take necessary safety measures, such as securing your campsite, keeping food away from wildlife, and carrying a first-aid kit. As with much of Southeast Asia, landmines and other unexploded ordinances are risky, so wandering in the scrub is not advisable.

Cambodia is home to various wild animals, including elephants and monkeys. Unfortunately, tigers were last seen in 2007. Although spotting wildlife can be an exciting part of your camping experience, it's essential to remember to keep a safe distance and avoid disturbing their natural habitats. Camping in Cambodia can be a unique and rewarding experience, allowing you to explore its stunning natural beauty and immerse yourself in its rich culture and history.

Campsites are limited, but here are a few

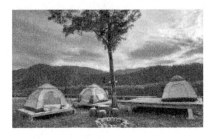

1 - Veal Chom Bang Camping
Unnamed Road, Chamcar Stung

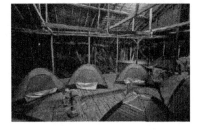

2 - The Scenery - Natural Campsite
See location 2 at the end of these regions' campsite pages.

3 - Shalom Valley Campsite
Krong Kaeb

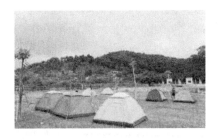

Laos may have a few more organized campsites than Cambodia, but neither region is well-equipped for camping tourism, unlike Thailand or Vietnam. Laos and Cambodia are much less developed in that regard. However, this doesn't mean camping is impossible; it requires creativity and patience. Being adventurous and even brave may come in handy. Fortunately, as with Laos, guesthouses and homestays in Cambodia are generally very affordable.

Vietnam

Camping

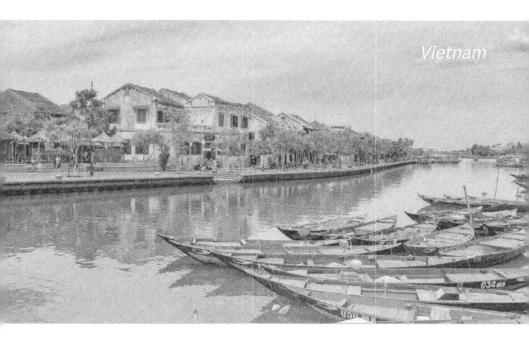

Vietnam

Vietnam is home to some of the most stunning natural landscapes in Southeast Asia, such as Ha Long Bay, the Mekong Delta, and the rice paddies of Sapa. Camping in these areas can provide a unique perspective and a chance to immerse oneself fully in nature.

Camping in Vietnam offers an opportunity to experience the country's rich cultural heritage. Local villages and communities have unique customs, traditions, and ways of life that can be fascinating to learn about and experience firsthand. There are various camping options available, such as beach camping, mountain camping, and forest camping. Each option offers a unique experience and an opportunity to explore different parts.

Camping in Vietnam can be an affordable way to explore the country, especially compared to other forms of accommodation. This makes it a popular option for backpackers, cyclists and budget travellers.

Many camping locations in Vietnam offer opportunities for adventure activities such as hiking, kayaking, and rock climbing. These activities can add an extra level of excitement and challenge to a camping trip in Vietnam. Camping provides a unique and immersive travel experience that combines natural beauty, cultural discovery, and adventure.

Campsites are numerous in the north and south

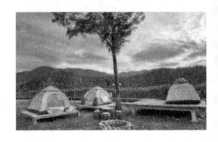

1 - Son Tinh Camp 3
Thôn Muồng Cháu, Ba Vì, Hà Nội

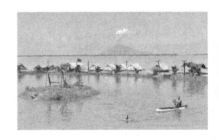

2 - Nhà Của Ba Campsite
Thị, Trung Lương, Phù Cát, Bình Định,

3 - Đồng Sến Farmstays
Dầu Tiếng District, Binh Duong

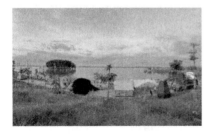

4 - Mada Lakeview Camping
Vĩnh Cửu, Đồng Nai

5 - PineForest Camping Đà Lạt
Phường 4, Thành phố Đà Lạt, Lâm Đồng

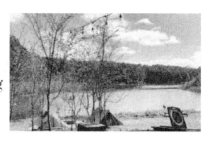

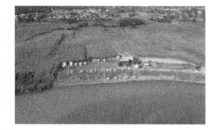

6 - Làng Mê
Hòa Vang, Đà Nẵng 50810

7 - Ham Lon Lake Campsite
Thôn, Thanh Hà, Sóc Sơn, Hà Nội

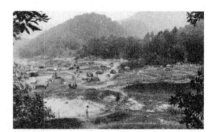

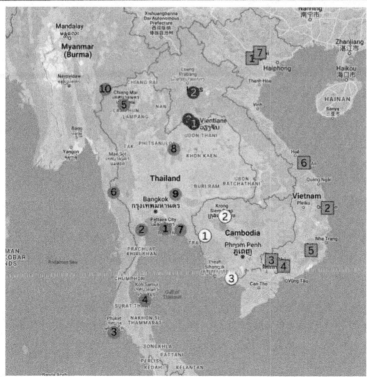

Thailand, Laos, Cambodia, Vietnam, campsite numbers on map

Wild Camping Pros & Cons

It is a great feeling to get off the road and camp in a field, forest, patch of unused ground, or even jungle. However, wild camping in Southeast Asia may differ from the West.

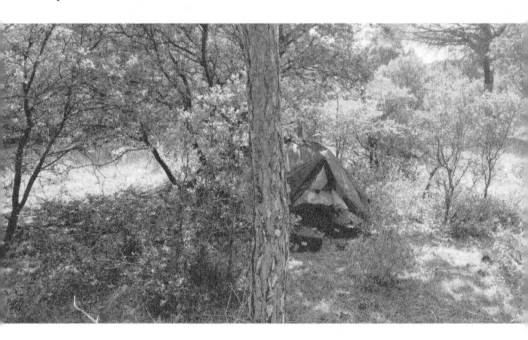

Wild camping in Southeast Asia can provide a distinct and exhilarating experience, but it has advantages and disadvantages. Below are a few to keep in mind:

Cons

Landmines: It is worth noting that Southeast Asia is a diverse region comprising several countries, each with its distinct characteristics and circumstances. However, landmines have been an issue in various parts of Southeast Asia, presenting a hazard to individuals in the region.

One of the most renowned instances of landmines in Southeast Asia is in Cambodia, where landmines were extensively deployed during the civil war in the 1970s and 1980s. Despite significant efforts by the government and international organizations to clear these landmines, they still pose a threat in some regions, including certain rural areas where camping or hiking may occur.

Apart from Cambodia, landmines have been deployed in Vietnam and Laos, during conflicts. Although these countries have made headway in removing landmines, certain regions still present a danger.

Researching the area you plan to visit and taking appropriate measures to ensure your safety is crucial. These may involve sticking to designated trails or areas, avoiding unfamiliar or suspicious objects, and seeking advice or guidance from local authorities. Additionally, it is vital to recognise the signs of landmines and report any suspected or unexploded ordnance.

Wild animals: The region harbours wildlife that can threaten humans. However, the degree of concern you should have will depend on various factors, such as your travel destination, the activities you plan to participate in, and the precautions you take.

If you plan to go trekking or camping in a remote area, you should be aware of the local wildlife and take precautions to avoid encounters. This might include avoiding hiking alone, making noise to alert animals to your presence, and storing food in a secure container to avoid attracting animals.

Seek advice from local authorities and guides who are familiar with the area. Additionally, it is vital to adhere to basic safety precautions, such as refraining from feeding or approaching wild animals, respecting their space and natural habitats, and seeking medical attention immediately if bitten or scratched by an animal. With the proper precautions and common sense, you can safely relish the region's numerous natural attractions.

Insects and creepy crawlies: Southeast Asia hosts a variety of insects, some of which can pose a threat to humans. Mosquitoes are prevalent and can carry malaria, dengue fever, and Zika virus. To prevent mosquito-borne illnesses, applying insect repellent when required is essential. If you don't mind having them, consider getting recommended vaccinations.

Safety and legality: Wild camping may not always be lawful in certain areas and you could encounter problems with the authorities in some areas. More likely, the authorities would be considering your safety than being jobsworths. In addition, when wild camping, you may have to forego numerous amenities you might take for granted in a hotel or hostel, such as running water, electricity, and access to toilets or showers.

Environmental impact: Wild camping can significantly impact the environment, and it is crucial to practice responsible camping by leaving no trace to reduce your impact on the local ecosystem.

Pros

Freedom and Flexibility: Wild camping lets you explore the great outdoors and plan your itinerary without sometimes worrying about finding accommodation. There's nothing quite like absorbing the sounds of a new environment throughout the night, including animal noises, wind and weather, and every snapping of a twig or rustle of leaves.

Cost: Wild camping is typically more cost-effective than staying in a hotel or hostel, making it a preferable choice for budget travellers. However, some cyclists embark on their journey with insufficient funds to comfortably complete their trip without relying on the kindness of strangers. In such cases, wild camping may not be an option but a necessity. Luckily, the people of Southeast Asia are amiable, and though they may live hand-to-mouth, they are often willing to provide floor space or shelter for those on a tight budget.

<u>Immersion in nature:</u> Camping in the wilderness can be a distinctive and engaging experience, providing an opportunity to have a closer look at the wildlife and environment. Southeast Asia is famous for its diverse and awe-inspiring landscape and nature. The region comprises the following countries: Brunei, Cambodia, East Timor, Indonesia, Laos, Malaysia, Myanmar, the Philippines, Singapore, Thailand, and Vietnam.

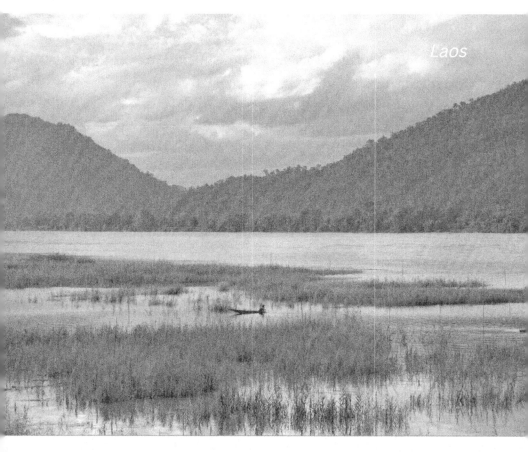

Laos

Southeast Asia prides itself on being home to some of the world's most magnificent coral reefs and beaches, celebrated for their immaculate white sands, crystal-clear waters, and awe-inspiring sunsets. The Similan Islands in Thailand are a famous group of islands in the Andaman Sea. The area is renowned for its crystal-clear waters, diverse marine life, and colourful coral reefs, making it a popular destination for snorkelling and diving enthusiasts.

The region boasts several prominent rivers, such as the Mekong and Red Rivers, which provide crucial habitats for various plant and animal species. Consequently, the landscape and nature are distinguished by diversity and beauty, making the region a sought-after destination for nature enthusiasts and adventure seekers.

For many cyclists, the advantages of wild camping in Southeast Asia surpass the disadvantages, and it is easy to understand why.

Anticipate frequent rain throughout the night most times of the year, with thunderstorms and flooding being common. Heat and humidity can sometimes cause even the most resilient individuals to feel like giving up. However, returning home with such experiences is priceless.

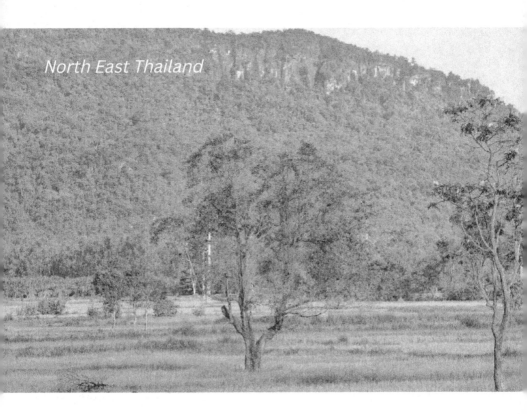

North East Thailand

Guesthouses & Other Places To Stay

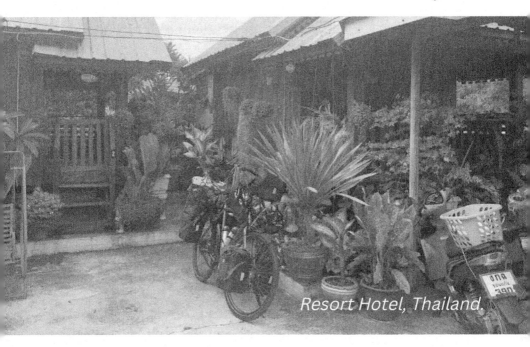

Resort Hotel, Thailand.

Campsites in the West can frequently be significantly more costly than homestays or guesthouses in Southeast Asia. Given the often harsh weather conditions and the prevalence of wild animals and insects in Southeast Asia, staying safe and dry in a building is a preferable alternative. After a hot day of travelling, taking a shower and enjoying some air conditioning are refreshing and can prepare most travellers for another adventure.

The first thing many people do when searching for accommodation is to look out for a sign outside a house or building that reads Wi-Fi/24-7 or something similar. This is a clear indication; a brief knock on the door will confirm whether it is a good place for you.

It is also crucial to note that many low-budget places are used for short-term entertainment. It is common to find packets of condoms in a dish in the room, and single male travellers may be asked if they require such entertainment. Don't be disheartened; brush it off and ask for the local beer.

The cleanliness in some very low-budget places could be better, and the adage 'you get what you pay for' also applies in Southeast Asia. Bugs can be a nuisance, so it's a good idea to spray the room with insect repellent and return an hour later. Geckos are harmless, and many rooms have one or two as residents. However, they can be noisy, making loud croaking and clicking noises throughout the night, which can be bothersome. Leaving a light on is a simple solution that often stops them and other bugs from coming out.

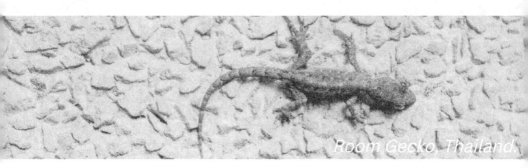
Room Gecko, Thailand.

Depending on your budget and preferences, there are several ways to find accommodation. Websites such as Booking.com, Agoda, and Airbnb enable you to search for accommodations based on your budget and location. You can filter results by price range, location, and accommodation, such as hotels, hostels, guesthouses, etc. If not, you can use the services of a travel agent to help you find places to stay. Travel agents have access to a broad range of accommodation options and can assist you in finding a place that meets your needs and budget.

Local guides or residents familiar with the area can also suggest accommodations not listed on online booking sites. You can also seek recommendations on travel forums or social media groups dedicated to travel in the region. Lastly, if you're comfortable with a degree of uncertainty, you can walk around an area where you're interested in staying and look for signs or advertisements for accommodations. This approach can be hit-or-miss but may lead you to discover hidden gems.

A Temple Guest

Visitors, including tourists, can generally enter temples during opening hours to pay respects, make offerings, or explore the site. However, staying overnight is typically reserved for those participating in meditation or other spiritual practices.

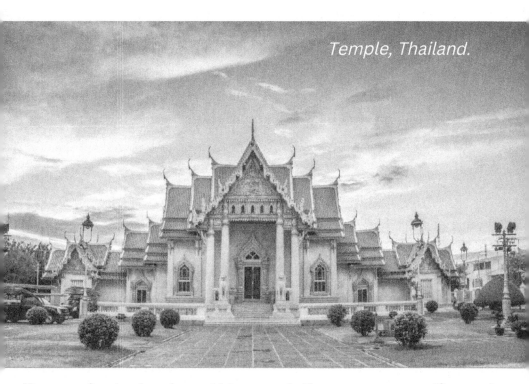

Temple, Thailand.

You can often book a place within a temple if you contact a specific temple beforehand. However, due to language barriers, many prefer to turn up on the day. Once you have chosen a temple, you can contact them directly to ask about their policies and availability. You can usually find contact information for the temple on its website or social media pages. Strangely, many temples have such web-based information.

When you contact the temple, explain your intentions for staying there, such as participating in meditation or other spiritual practices. Be respectful and mindful of the temple's rules and traditions.

Once you have permission, arrange your stay and any necessary details with the temple staff. They may ask you to bring your bedding or to follow specific guidelines during your visit. It's essential to remember that temples are places of worship and spiritual practice, so visitors should respect the temple's customs and traditions. Dress modestly and remove your shoes before entering—any sacred areas. Additionally, you should follow any rules or guidelines the temple staff provides during your stay.

It's not unheard of that after spending a night or two at a temple in Southeast Asia, some people have decided to become followers and leave their old lives behind. So, ensure your estate is in order before heading out there. That last part regarding getting your estate in order was intended to be humorous, maybe.

Hostels

Hostels can be found throughout Southeast Asia. Southeast Asia is a popular destination for budget travellers, cyclists, backpackers, and digital nomads, and there are many hostels to choose from. Hostels can be found in popular tourist destinations such as Bangkok, Chiang Mai, Ho Chi Minh City, Siem Reap, and many others. Southeast Asian hostels are often very affordable and offer a range of accommodation options, from dormitory beds to private rooms. Some hostels also have social spaces, such as bars or communal kitchens, which make them great places to meet other travellers. Southeast Asia is great for finding affordable and comfortable hostel accommodations while travelling, and secure bike storage is often available.

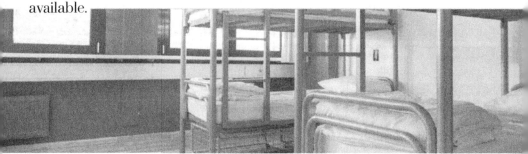

Thailand

Thailand is a popular destination for backpackers and budget travellers, and many hostels exist nationwide. These are just a few examples of the many hostels available in Thailand. When choosing a hostel, read reviews, check amenities, and consider location and price.

Mad Monkey Hostel in Bangkok: This hostel is located in the heart of Bangkok's backpacker district, Khao San Road. The hostel has a lively atmosphere, with a rooftop bar, pool table, and organized social events.

Slumber Party Hostel in Krabi: This hostel is in Ao Nang, a popular beach town in southern Thailand. They offer dormitory beds and private rooms and have a fun and sociable atmosphere with a bar and organized activities.

The Yard Hostel in Bangkok: This hostel is located in the trendy Ari neighbourhood of Bangkok and offers both dormitory beds and private rooms. The hostel has a garden and outdoor seating area and is known for its relaxed and welcoming atmosphere.

Lub d Hostel in Chiang Mai: This hostel is located in the heart of Chiang Mai and offers modern and stylish accommodations with comfortable beds and social spaces. The hostel has a bar, cafe, and co-working space, making it an excellent option for digital nomads.

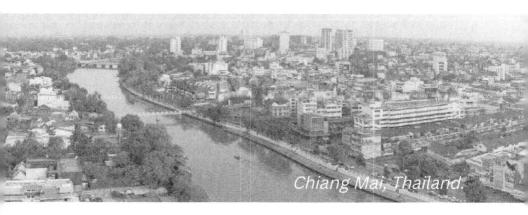

Chiang Mai, Thailand.

Laos

Staying in hostels is a popular option for cyclists and other travellers in Laos. These hostels offer a range of accommodations, from dormitory-style rooms to private rooms. They also provide amenities like free Wi-Fi, breakfast, and tour booking services. Staying in hostels can be a great way to meet other travellers and explore Laos on a budget. Some examples of hostels in Laos include:

Downtown Backpackers Hostel in Vientiane: A popular hostel located in the capital city of Laos, Vientiane. The hostel offers dormitory-style rooms and private rooms. The hostel is in the city centre, providing access to many of Vientiane's main attractions.

The Siamese Cat Hostel: The hostel is located in the heart of Luang Prabang, within walking distance of many of the town's main attractions, such as the night market and the Royal Palace Museum. The hostel offers free Wi-Fi, a communal kitchen, and a rooftop terrace with a bar and restaurant.

The Funky Monkey Hostel: The hostel is close to many of Pakse's main attractions, such as the Pakse night market and the Mekong River. The hostel offers free Wi-Fi, a bar and restaurant, and a rooftop terrace with great city views.

Don Det Hostel: This is a popular hostel located on the island of Don Det in the 4000 Islands region. The hostel is peaceful and scenic, with beautiful views of the Mekong River and easy access to the island's many natural attractions, such as waterfalls and swimming spots.

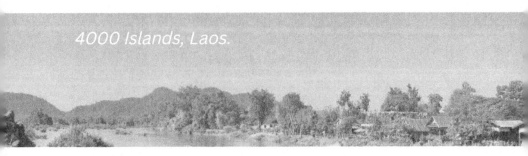

4000 Islands, Laos.

Cambodia

Staying in hostels in Cambodia can be a budget-friendly and social way to explore the country. Hostels in Cambodia are generally located in major cities and tourist destinations, such as Phnom Penh, Siem Reap, and Sihanoukville. In addition, hostels are often centrally located, making it easy for guests to explore the local attractions and cuisine.

Mad Monkey Hostel: This hostel has Phnom Penh and Siem Reap locations and is known for its lively and social atmosphere. It offers a variety of room types, including dorms and private rooms, and has a bar, restaurant, and pool.

The Big Easy Hostel: Located in the heart of Phnom Penh, offers clean and comfortable accommodations with a laid-back atmosphere. It has a rooftop bar and restaurant and offers free Wi-Fi and a range of tours and activities.

Hometown Hostel: This hostel in Battambang offers a range of room types, including private rooms and dorms, and has a garden and outdoor seating area. It offers free Wi-Fi and organizes activities such as city tours and bike rentals.

Footprint Hostel: Located in Sihanoukville, Footprint Hostel offers dormitory-style accommodations focusing on sustainability and community. It has a rooftop terrace and bar and provides a range of activities, such as beach cleanups and local tours.

Sihanoukville, Cambodia.

Vietnam

Vietnam has a range of hostels catering to budget travellers. Hostels in Vietnam offer clean and affordable accommodations, making them popular for cyclists and backpackers. Many hostels also provide social spaces and organized activities, making it easy for travellers to meet and connect.

Central Backpackers Hostel, Hanoi: This is a popular hostel located in the heart of the Old Quarter. The hostel also has a rooftop bar and lounge and is a great place to socialise with other travellers and enjoy the city views.

Saigon Backpackers Hostel: This is a well-known hostel in the heart of Ho Chi Minh City's backpacker district. The hostel offers both private rooms and dormitories, all of which are air-conditioned and come with comfortable beds.

Hue Backpackers Hostel: This is a popular hostel in the city of Hue, Vietnam. The hostel is in the city's heart, close to many historical landmarks and attractions.

Cozy Nook Hostel: This is a charming hostel in Da La. The hostel is conveniently located close to the city centre, making it an excellent base for exploring Da Lat.

Mui Ne Backpacker Village, Mui Ne: This hostel offers affordable dormitory-style accommodation with basic amenities such as shared bathrooms, communal areas, and free Wi-Fi.

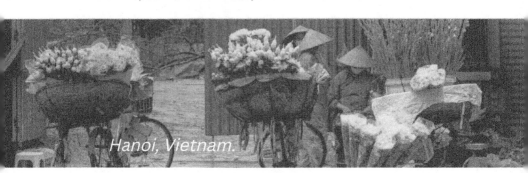

Hanoi, Vietnam.

CHAPTER NINE
Popular Routes

We have already explored why cycle touring in Southeast Asia is a fantastic experience. Next, let's delve into popular routes across our four regions: Thailand, Laos, Cambodia, and Vietnam. We will look at both day routes around popular tourist spots and longer routes that may take several days or much longer to complete. Also, we'll include links to Google Maps where possible, allowing you to study the routes online. Although we cannot guarantee the longevity of these links, they may prove helpful while they are available. Some maps may be set for walking or cycling, but both will be great for cycling. More often than not, the walking route is best for cycling.

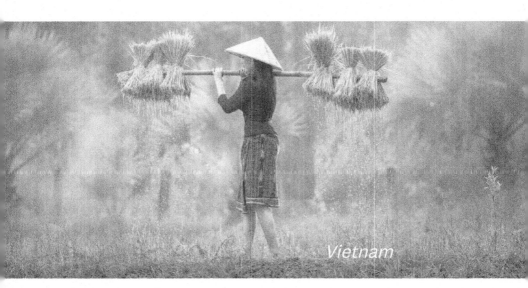

Vietnam

Thailand

Thailand is a popular cyclist destination, offering various cycle routes catering to different experiences and interests. Here are some popular cycle routes in Thailand:

<u>Mae Hong Son loop:</u> The Mae Hong Son Loop is a challenging and rewarding route that takes you through the northern mountains of Thailand. The route starts and ends in Chiang Mai and takes several days to complete. You will ride through stunning scenery, hill tribe villages, and winding mountain roads. The route also includes the Doi Inthanon National Park.

Mae Hong Son Loop - Distance 600km (373m)

Google Maps Web Link- t.ly/MaeHongSonLoop

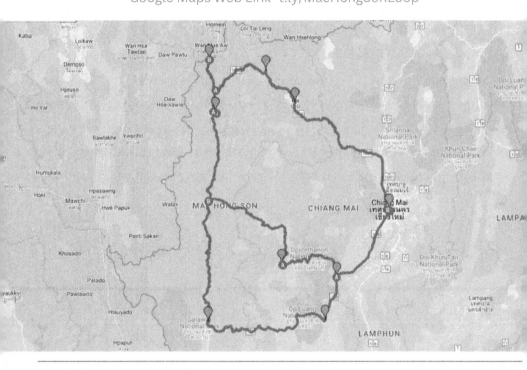

<u>Bangkok to Ayutthaya:</u> This is a popular day route that takes you from the bustling city of Bangkok to the historic city of Ayutthaya. The route follows the Chao Phraya River, passing through small towns, rural areas, and ancient temples. It is a flat, easy ride suitable for all experience levels.

Popular Routes

Bangkok to Ayutthaya - Distance 73km (45m)
Google Maps Web Link - t.ly/BangkokAyutthaya

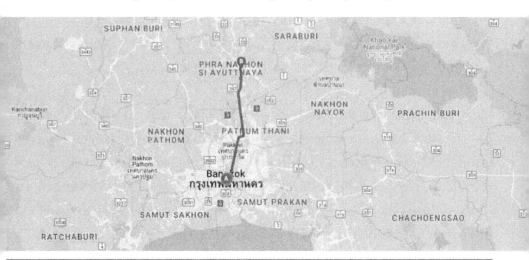

<u>Chiang Mai to Chiang Rai:</u> This is a longer route that can take several days to complete, but it is worth it for the stunning scenery and cultural experiences along the way. The route takes you through mountainous terrain, lush forests, and remote villages. In addition, you will have the opportunity to visit hill tribe communities, hot springs, and ancient temples.

Chiang Mai to Chiang Rai - Distance 184km (114m)
Google Maps Web Link - t.ly/ChiangMaiChiangRai

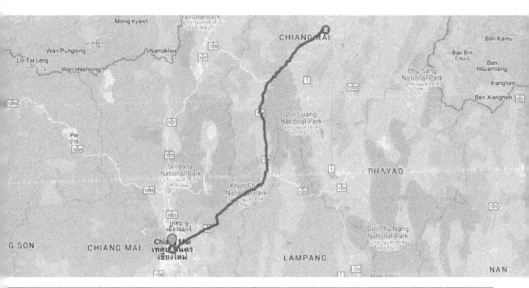

Great Isan Loop: This route is a long-distance/two-week loop that takes you through the northeastern region of Thailand, known as the country's breadbasket. Beginning and ending in Bangkok, it's an excellent route you can tweak for those who want a couple of weeks of adventurous cycling in the rural areas of Thailand that few cycle tourists explore.

On the Khorat Plateau, you'll ride along endless, gently winding roads passing through industrial areas, towns and villages, with few tourists around. The route takes you through field after field of rice paddies and wildlife reserves and offers days of cycling along the mighty Mekong River. If you occasionally get off some of the larger busy roads, you can expect to discover some hidden gems of tradition and culture.

Great Isan Loop - Distance 1912km (1188m)
Google Maps Web Link - t.ly/GreatIsanLoop

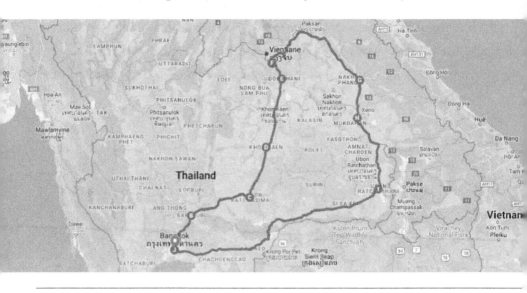

Bangkok to Phuket: This long-distance route can be started from Bangkok or the other way around, which many prefer. The route takes you through picturesque countryside, national parks, and charming beach towns such as Hua Hin and Krabi before concluding in Phuket. Along the way, you can experience stunning coastal views and immerse yourself in the local culture.

Bangkok to Phuket - Distance 951km (590m)
Google Maps Web Link - t.ly/BangkokPhuket

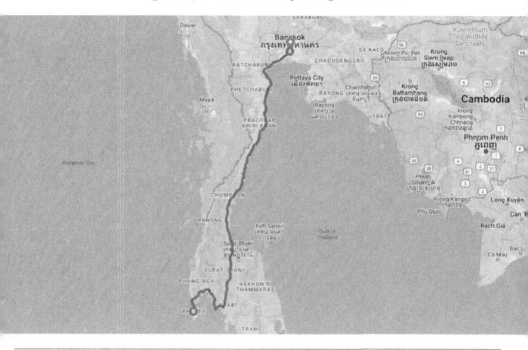

Chiang Mai to Bangkok: Starting in Chiang Mai, you'll ride through the lush countryside and mountainous regions of northern Thailand, passing through charming villages and towns. As you continue southward, you'll encounter the bustling city of Ayutthaya, which boasts an impressive array of historical sites and landmarks, including ancient ruins and ornate temples.

The journey's final stretch takes you through the flat terrain of central Thailand, passing through rice fields, orchards, and small towns. You'll finally reach Bangkok, one of Asia's most vibrant and exciting cities, where you can take in the sights and sounds of this bustling metropolis.

Whether you're an experienced cyclist or a first-time adventurer, cycling from Chiang Mai to Bangkok for a week or more is an unforgettable experience that will allow you to explore the heart and soul of Thailand.

Chiang Mai to Bangkok - Distance 677km (420m)

Google Maps Web Link - t.ly/ChiangMaiBangkok

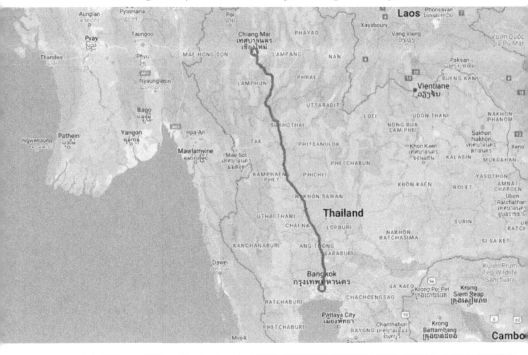

Bangkok to Trat: Cycling from Bangkok to Trat is an incredible adventure that takes you through Thailand's beautiful scenery and areas where many ex-pats have set up homes. The route begins in Bangkok, a bustling metropolis with a vibrant mix of culture and history. As you make your way eastward, you'll ride through idyllic countryside and small villages, where you'll have the opportunity to experience the local culture and hospitality.

As you continue cycling, you'll eventually reach Trat, a charming coastal town with beautiful beaches, clear waters, and a relaxed atmosphere. Along the way, you'll encounter numerous sights and experiences that make cycling from Bangkok to Trat unforgettable. This route has everything from the bustling streets of Bangkok to the idyllic countryside and beautiful coastline. Whether you're an experienced cyclist or a first-time adventurer, this route will leave a lasting impression.

Popular Routes

Bangkok to Trat - Distance 387km (240m)
Google Maps Web Link - t.ly/BangkokTrat

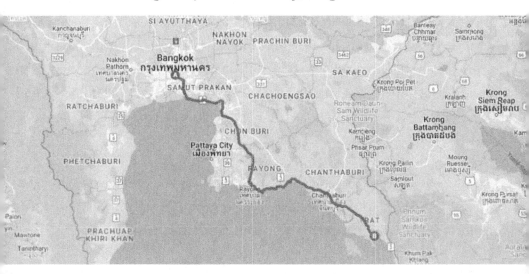

Bangkok to Kanchanaburi: This short route takes you westward from Bangkok to the famous River Kwai Bridge and the Hellfire Pass.

Bangkok to Kanchanaburi - Distance 138km (86m)
Google Maps Web Link - t.ly/BangkokKanchanaburi

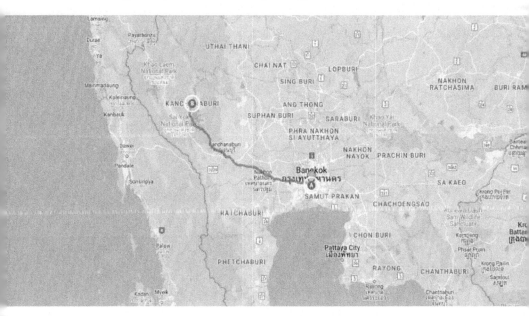

As with Thailand, the following routes in Laos, Cambodia, and Vietnam are great. However, most cycle tourists find that planning a route as they ride is the most rewarding way to explore Southeast Asia. Every turn can lead to surprises and adventures. Other cyclists prefer arranged tours, where they pay agents to plan their days, carry their gear, and even provide their meals. Each to their own, of course, as we are all different, and our rides are a personal choice that can be just as enjoyable as someone else's.

Laos

Cycling in Laos can be a rewarding and unforgettable experience for cyclists of all levels. Laos offers stunning scenery, friendly locals, and a rich cultural experience that can only be truly appreciated on a bicycle.

Vientiane to Pakse: This route takes you through the heart of Laos, including the UNESCO World Heritage site of Wat Phou, before reaching the bustling city of Pakse. Views of the Mekong River and over to Thailand can be had.

Vientiane to Pakse - Distance 666km (413m)
Google Maps Web Link - t.ly/VientianePakse

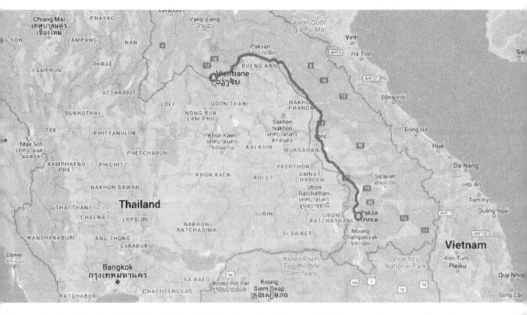

Luang Prabang to Vang Vieng: Luang Prabang, located in a valley at the meeting point of the Mekong and Nam Khan rivers, was once the capital of Luang Prabang Province in northern Laos. During your cycling adventure, you will pass through charming villages, verdant forests, and breathtaking limestone karst formations.

Luang Prabang to Vang Vieng - Distance 183km (113m)
Google Maps Web Link - t.ly/LuangPrabangVangVieng

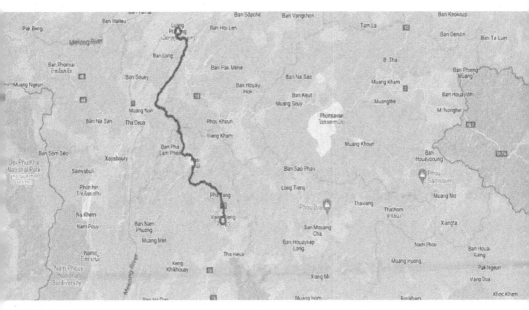

The Bolaven Plateau: The cooler temperatures and the higher altitude of the Bolaven Plateau will bring you blessed relief from the heat of Laos. Combine that with the many waterfalls in the region and the fact that this is Lao's central coffee region, and you have a great place to explore. Aside from waterfalls and coffee plantations, you'll find small villages teeming with local life, fresh food, and a lush jungle.

The Bolaven Plateau - Distance 316km (196m)
Google Maps Web Link - t.ly/TheBolavenPlateau

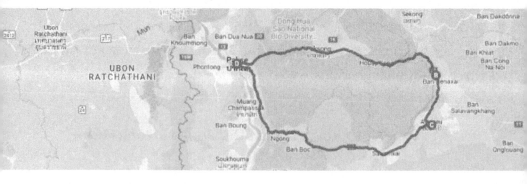

Vientiane to Phonsavan and the Plain of Jars Route: The Plain of Jars is a mysterious and fascinating region in central Laos known for its ancient stone jars. The route takes you through beautiful karst limestone formations, rice paddies, and traditional villages. You can start in Phonsavan and cycle north towards Muang Khoun. It is important to note that landmines remain in many areas in Laos, so care should be taken to stay within designated roads and tracks.

Plain of Jars - Distance 332km (206m)
Google Maps Web Link - t.ly/PlainOfJars

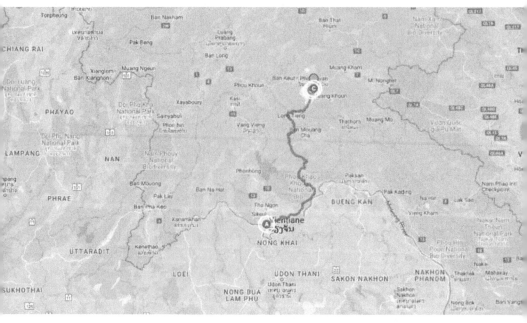

Cambodia

Bicycle touring in Cambodia can be a fantastic way to explore the country's stunning landscapes, rich culture, and friendly people. If you like it flat, you've got it; if you want some challenging hills, you've got that too.

Phnom Penh to Siem Reap: This route is a popular cycling tour in Cambodia. Depending on your pace and the number of stops, and the distance between the two cities, it can take around a week to complete. If you take certain roads, you may need a ferry crossing, which is enjoyable.

Phnom Penh to Siem Reap - Distance 303km (188m)
Google Maps Web Link - t.ly/PhnomPenhSiemReap

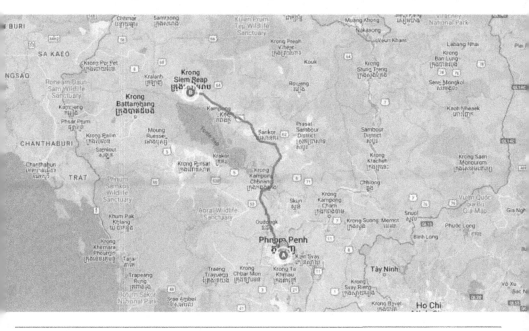

West to East Cambodia: This route is commonly chosen by travellers who want to cross Cambodia without encountering the popular tourist spots of Siem Reap and Angkor Wat. The journey involves passing through the border crossings of Krong Poi Pet, which borders Thailand, and Krong Bavet, which borders Vietnam and is close to Ho Chi Minh City, a city still referred to as Saigon by many locals. East to the west is the alternative, of course.

Cycling Southeast Asia

West to East Cambodia - Distance 548km (340m)

Google Maps Web Link - t.ly/WestToEastCambodia

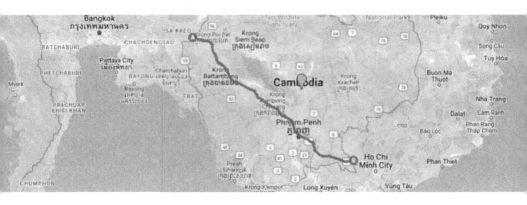

Angkor Wat Loop: The loop guides you through the temples of Angkor Wat. Starting from Siem Reap, the journey can take around an hour to cycle leisurely to the Angkor Wat temple, then to Phnom Bakheng Temple, Bayon Temple, Preah Khan Temple, Neak Poan, East Baray, and back to Siem Reap.

Angkor Wat Loop - Distance 38km (24m)

Google Maps Web Link - t.ly/AngkorWatLoop

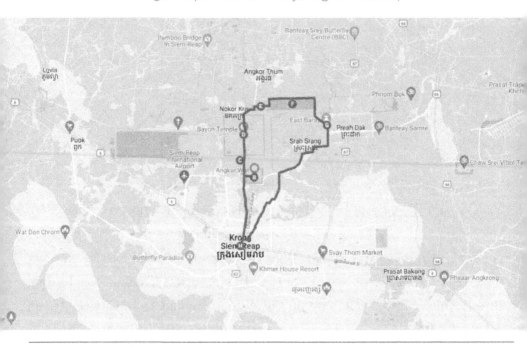

<u>Phnom Penh to Kampot:</u> This route takes you from the capital city of Phnom Penh to the coastal town of Kampot. You'll pass through scenic countryside, quaint villages, and historic sites along the way.

Phnom Penh to Kampot - Distance 147km (91m)
Google Maps Web Link - t.ly/PhnomPenhKampot

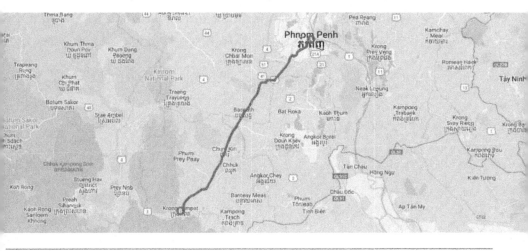

<u>Coastal Cambodia:</u> This is a picturesque journey along the coastline, with stops at delightful fishing villages, sandy beaches, and forests. Additionally, time permitting, you can take a detour into the Cardamom Mountains.

Coastal Cambodia - Distance 321km (200m)
Google Maps Web Link - t.ly/CoastalCambodia

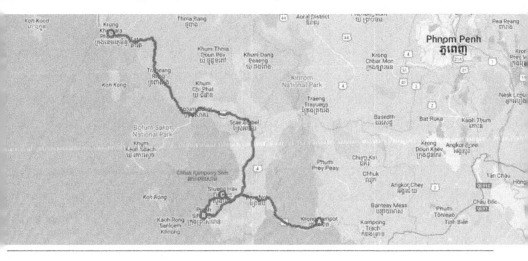

Vietnam

Vietnam is scenic, with mountainous terrain and a lengthy coastline, including the breathtaking Mekong Delta. This makes it an ideal destination for cycle touring enthusiasts.

Hanoi to Ho Chi Minh City: The journey will lead you through the stunning Vietnamese countryside, with stops at historical landmarks, traditional villages, and vibrant cities. Completing this route could take several weeks.

Hanoi to Ho Chi Minh City - Distance 1800km (1118m)
Google Maps Web Link - t.ly/HanoiHoChiMinh

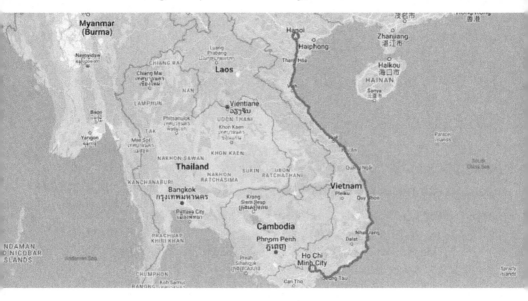

Ho Chi Minh Trail: It was not a single road or route but a complex network of roads, footpaths, and waterways spanning Vietnam, Laos, and Cambodia. It served as a supply line for the North Vietnamese Army and was a constantly evolving system of supply routes, adapting to the ever-changing circumstances on the ground. The trail traversed through remote and challenging terrain, such as mountains, forests, and swamps, and was often heavily guarded by the North Vietnamese Army. If you cycle almost anywhere in Vietnam, you will likely encounter or ride along various sections of this vast and intricate trail. We have kept within Vietnam for this.

Ho Chi Minh Trail - Hanoi to Ho Chi Minh City - 1860km (1156m)
Google Maps Web Link - t.ly/HoChiMinhTrail

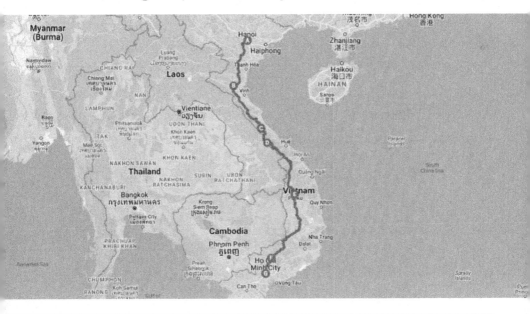

Hanoi Sapa Loop: The Hanoi Sapa Loop is a challenging ride leading you to the region's high hills and mountains. While the sights can be spectacular, the journey can be highly demanding for many. On the way out, you'll ride along the Red River. Due to the limited number of hotels along the way, you may need warm camping equipment.

Hanoi Sapa Loop - 726km (451m)
Google Maps Web Link - t.ly/HanoiSapaLoop

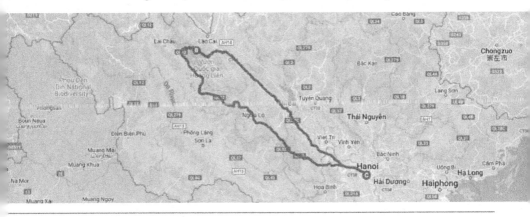

<u>Mekong Delta Loop:</u> Cycling the Mekong Delta is a popular activity among tourists visiting Vietnam. The Mekong Delta is a vast area in southern Vietnam where the Mekong River flows into the South China Sea. It is a beautiful region with fertile land, diverse wildlife, and a rich cultural heritage.

As you can expect from such low-lying land, it's flat. You'll cross many waterways over small bridges and by ferries.

Mekong Delta Loop - Distance 460km (285m)

Google Maps Web Link - t.ly/HanoiHoChiMinh

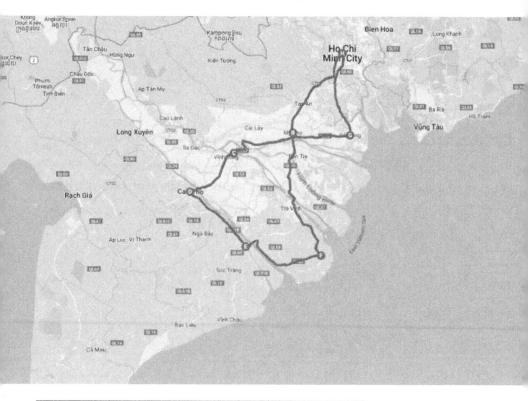

CHAPTER TEN
Seasons

Southeast Asia is a region with diverse climates and landscapes and has a range of different seasons and weather patterns throughout the year. Here is a brief overview of the seasons in Southeast Asia:

Dry season: The dry season typically runs from December to April in most Southeast Asia, although the exact timing can vary depending on the location. During the dry season, temperatures are generally hot and sunny, with lower daily rainfall. This makes it a popular time to visit the beaches and islands of Southeast Asia, as well as to explore the cities and cultural attractions.

Wet season: The wet season generally runs from May to November in most parts of Southeast Asia, although the exact timing can vary depending on the location. During the wet season, temperatures are generally cooler and there is more rainfall, which can lead to flooding and other weather-related issues. However, the wet season can also be a beautiful time to visit, as the lush vegetation and waterfalls are at their most vibrant.

Monsoon season: Some parts of Southeast Asia experience a monsoon season with heavy rainfall and strong winds. The monsoon season can vary depending on the location but generally runs from June to September in most parts of the region.

<u>High season:</u> The high season generally corresponds with the dry season, the busiest time for tourism in Southeast Asia. This is when prices for accommodations and activities are typically higher, and crowds can be larger. However, the high season also offers the best weather and the most reliable travel conditions.

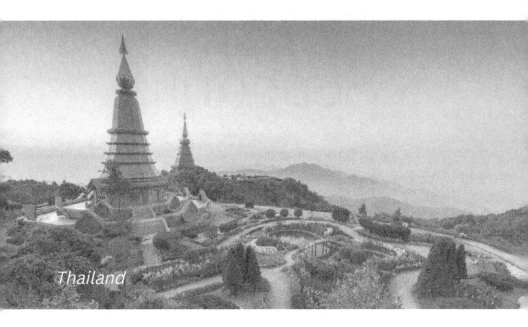

Thailand

As with any destination, the weather in Southeast Asia can often be unpredictable upon arrival. The promised warm sunshine may be nowhere to be seen, or the cool sea breezes may feel more like hurricane-force winds. All we can do is hope for the best.

It can be challenging to predict the weather forecast for each location in each country, as weather patterns can vary slightly. However, the following tables provide approximate weather patterns based on the central parts of each country. Remember that temperatures may be slightly colder the farther north you go and warmer the farther south you go. Similarly, areas farther north may experience more rainfall, while areas farther south may be drier. While these charts we have created, based on historical data, can only provide an idea, we hope they help you plan your trip.

Seasons

Thailand

Chiang Mai - Northern Thailand

Month	Average low (°C)	Average Low (°F)	Average high (°C)	Average High (°F)	Precip. (mm)	Precip. (inches)	Precip. days
Jan	14.9	48.8	29.8	85.6	4.2	0.16	1
Feb	16.2	61.1	32.7	90.8	8.9	0.35	1
Mar	19.5	67.1	35.2	95.3	17.8	0.7	2
Apr	22.9	73.2	36.5	97.7	57.3	2.25	7
May	23.8	74.8	34.2	93.5	162	6.37	15
Jun	24	75.2	32.7	90.8	124.5	4.88	17
Jul	23.9	75	31.8	89.2	140.2	5.51	19
Aug	23.7	74.6	31.5	88.7	216.9	8.53	21
Sept	23.2	73.7	31.7	89	211.4	8.32	18
Oct	22.2	71.9	31.4	88.5	117.6	4.62	12
Nov	19.2	66.5	30.1	86.1	53.9	2.12	5
Dec	15.7	60.2	28.6	83.4	15.9	0.62	1
Totals	20.8	68.5	32.2	89.8	1130.6	44.43	118
	Daily/Av	Daily/Av	Daily/Av	Daily/Av	Year	Year	Year

Bangkok - Central Thailand

Month	Average Low (°C)	Average Low (°F)	Average High (°C)	Average High (°F)	Precip. (mm)	Precip. (inches)	Precip. days
Jan	22.6	72.6	32.5	90.5	13.3	0.52	2
Feb	24.4	75.2	33.3	91.9	20	0.78	2
Mar	25.9	78.6	34.3	93.7	42.1	1.65	4
Apr	26.9	80.4	35.4	95.7	91.4	3.59	7
May	26.3	79.3	34.4	93.9	247.7	9.75	16
Jun	26.1	78.9	33.6	92.4	157.1	6.18	16
Jul	25.7	78.2	33.2	91.7	175.1	6.89	17
Aug	25.5	77.9	32.9	91.2	219.3	8.63	19
Sept	25	77	32.8	91	334.2	10.10	21
Oct	24.8	76.6	32.6	90.6	292.1	11.5	17
Nov	23.9	75	32.4	90.3	49.5	1.94	6
Dec	22	71	31.7	89	6.3	0.24	1
Totals	24.9	76.7	33.3	91.8	1648.2	64.83	128
	Daily/Av	Daily/Av	Daily/Av	Daily/Av	Year	Year	Year

Surat Thani - Southern Thailand

Month	Average low (°C)	Average Low (°F)	Average high (°C)	Average High (°F)	Precip. (mm)	Precip. (inches)	Precip. days
Jan	24.2	75.5	29	84.2	86.2	3.39	11
Feb	25	77	29.4	84.9	54.4	2.14	6
Mar	25.6	78	30.6	87	80.8	3.18	6
Apr	26.1	78.9	32	89.6	83.1	3.27	9
May	25.7	78.2	32.6	90.6	155.9	6.13	16
Jun	25.5	77.9	32.5	90.5	124.1	4.88	14
Jul	25.1	77.1	32.2	89.9	116.3	4.57	14
Aug	25.2	77.3	32.1	89.7	110.9	4.36	15
Sept	24.8	76.6	31.7	89	121.7	4.79	16
Oct	24.3	75.7	30.5	86.9	309.8	12.19	20
Nov	24.1	75.3	29.6	85.2	506.6	19.94	20
Dec	23.9	75	29.2	84.5	210.3	8.27	14
Totals	24.9	76.8	30.95	87.6	1960.1	77.11	161
	Daily/Av	Daily/Av	Daily/Av	Daily/Av	Year	Year	Year

Laos

Since Laos is landlocked and relatively small, we have compiled its climate information into a single chart. The southern regions will likely experience slightly warmer temperatures than the central areas, while the northern parts can be slightly cooler.

Month	Average low (°C)	Average Low (°F)	Average high (°C)	Average High (°F)	Precip. (mm)	Precip. (inches)	Precip. days
Jan	16.4	61.5	28.4	83.1	7.5	0.29	1
Feb	18.5	65.3	30.3	86.5	13	0.51	2
Mar	21.5	76.1	33	91.4	33.7	1.32	4
Apr	23.8	74.8	34.3	93.7	84.9	3.34	8
May	24.6	76.2	33	91.4	245.8	9.67	15
Jun	24.9	76.8	31.9	89.4	279.8	11	18
Jul	24.7	76.4	31.3	88.3	272.3	10.7	20
Aug	24.6	76.2	30.8	87.4	334.6	13.17	21
Sept	24.1	75.3	30.9	87.6	297.3	11.7	17
Oct	22.9	73.2	30.8	87.4	78	3	9
Nov	19.3	66.7	29.8	85.6	11.1	0.43	2
Dec	16.7	62	28.1	82.5	2.5	0.09	1
Totals	21.8	71.7	31	87.8	1660.5	65.22	118
	Daily/Av	Daily/Av	Daily/Av	Daily/Av	Year	Year	Year

Cambodia

Since Cambodia's dimensions have a maximum width of about 555km (345m) from east to west and a maximum height of about 450km (280m) from north to south, we have compiled its climate information into a single chart. Coast and highlands can be cooler.

Month	Average low (°C)	Average Low (°F)	Average high (°C)	Average High (°F)	Precip. (mm)	Precip. (inches)	Precip. days
Jan	21.8	71.2	31.6	88.8	12.1	0.47	1
Feb	22.8	73	33.2	91.7	6.6	0.25	1
Mar	24.3	75.7	34.6	94.2	34.8	1.37	3
Apr	25.5	77.9	35.3	95.5	78.8	3.1	7
May	25.6	78	34.8	94.6	118.2	4.65	16
Jun	24.9	76.8	33.8	92.8	145	5.7	17
Jul	24.9	76.8	32.9	91.2	162.1	6.38	18
Aug	24.6	76.2	32.7	90.8	182.7	7.19	18
Sept	24.3	75.7	32.2	89.9	270.9	10.66	21
Oct	24.2	75.5	31.4	88.5	248.1	9.76	19
Nov	23.2	73.7	31.1	87.9	120.5	4.74	10
Dec	21.9	71.4	30.8	87.4	32.1	1.26	4
Totals	24	75.1	32.9	91.1	1411.9	55.53	135
	Daily/Av	Daily/Av	Daily/Av	Daily/Av	Year	Year	Year

Vietnam
Hanoi - Northern Vietnam

Month	Average low (°C)	Average Low (°F)	Average high (°C)	Average High (°F)	Precip. (mm)	Precip. (inches)	Precip. days
Jan	13.7	56.6	19.3	66.7	18.6	0.73	8
Feb	15	59	19.9	67.8	26.2	1.03	11
Mar	18.1	64.5	22.8	73	43.8	1.72	15
Apr	21.4	70.5	27	80.6	90.1	3.54	13
May	24.3	75.7	31.5	88.7	188.5	7.42	14
Jun	25.8	78.4	32.6	90.6	239.9	9.44	15
Jul	26.1	78.9	32.9	91.2	288.2	11.34	16
Aug	25.7	78.2	31.9	89.4	318	12.51	17
Sept	24.7	76.4	30.9	87.6	265.4	10.44	14
Oct	21.9	71.4	28.6	83.4	130.7	5.14	9
Nov	18.5	65.3	25.2	77.3	43.4	1.7	7
Dec	15.3	59.5	21.8	71.2	23.4	0.92	6
Totals	20.8	69.5	27	80.6	1676.2	65.93	145
	Daily/Av	Daily/Av	Daily/Av	Daily/Av	Year	Year	Year

Da Nang - Central Vietnam

Month	Average low (°C)	Average Low (°F)	Average high (°C)	Average High (°F)	Precip. (mm)	Precip. (inches)	Precip. days
Jan	18.5	65.3	24.8	76.6	96.2	3.78	14
Feb	19.8	67.6	26.1	78.9	33	1.29	7
Mar	21.5	70.7	28.7	83.6	22.4	0.88	5
Apr	23.3	73.9	31	87.8	26.9	1.05	6
May	24.9	76.8	33.4	92.1	62.6	2.46	9
Jun	25.5	77.9	33.9	93	87.1	3.42	8
Jul	25.3	77.5	34.3	93.7	85.6	3.37	9
Aug	25.5	77.9	33.9	93	103	4.05	11
Sept	24.1	75.3	31.5	88.7	349.7	13.76	15
Oct	23.2	73.7	29.6	85.2	612.8	24.12	21
Nov	21.6	70.8	27	80.6	366.2	14.41	21
Dec	19.3	66.7	24.9	76.8	199	7.83	19
Totals	22.7	72.8	29.9	85.8	2044.5	80.42	145
	Daily/Av	Daily/Av	Daily/Av	Daily/Av	Year	Year	Year

Ho Chi Minh City - Southern Vietnam

Month	Average low (°C)	Average Low (°F)	Average high (°C)	Average High (°F)	Precip. (mm)	Precip. (inches)	Precip. days
Jan	21.1	69.9	31.6	88.8	13.8	0.54	2
Feb	22.5	72.5	32.9	91.2	4.1	0.16	1
Mar	24.4	76.2	33.9	93	10.5	0.41	2
Apr	25.8	78.4	34.6	94.2	50.4	1.98	5
May	25.2	77.3	34	93.2	218.4	8.59	18
Jun	24.6	76.2	32.4	90.3	311.7	12.27	19
Jul	24.3	75.7	32	89.6	293.7	11.56	23
Aug	24.3	75.7	31.8	89.2	269.8	10.62	22
Sept	24.4	75.9	31.3	88.3	327.1	12.87	23
Oct	23.9	75	31.2	88.1	266.7	10.5	21
Nov	22.8	73	31	87.8	116.5	4.58	12
Dec	21.4	75.5	30.8	87.8	48.3	1.9	7
Totals	23.7	75.1	32.2	90.1	1931	75.98	155
	Daily/Av	Daily/Av	Daily/Av	Daily/Av	Year	Year	Year

We will re-examine the charts and adopt a fresh perspective on the weather and conditions in the four highlighted nations. Naturally, the well-known phrase "as changeable as the weather" applies to Southeast Asia, just like other parts of the world.

Thailand

The climate in Thailand varies throughout the year, so selecting the right time for your visit is essential. Generally, the most suitable time to travel is during the cool, dry season, which extends from November to February.

In the north, including Chiang Mai and Chiang Rai, the climate features three distinct seasons: a cool, dry period from November to February, a hot season from March to May, and a rainy season from June to October. The ideal time to explore this region is between November and February when the weather is cooler and more comfortable.

Central Thailand, encompassing cities like Bangkok and Ayutthaya, experiences a tropical monsoon climate. The hot season occurs from March to May, followed by the rainy season from June to October, and the cool, dry season from November to February. The most favourable time to visit this area is during the cool season when the temperatures are more pleasant, and the humidity is lower.

Southern Thailand, including popular destinations like Phuket, Krabi, and Koh Samui, has a tropical climate with high humidity. The region is split into two distinct weather patterns: the East Coast experiences its wet season from September to December, while the West Coast's rainy season occurs from April to October. The best time to visit the east coast is from January to March, and for the west coast, the ideal period is from November to March.

To make the most of your Thai adventure, carefully consider the region's climate and aim to travel during the cool, dry season for the most enjoyable weather conditions.

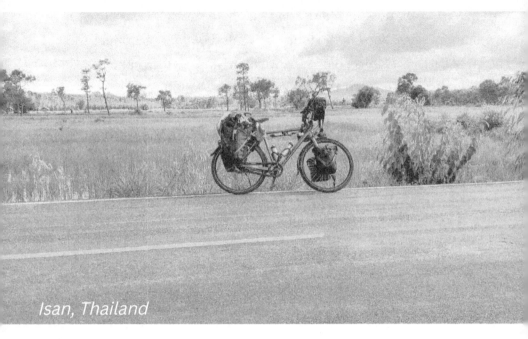

Isan, Thailand

Laos

The climate in Laos varies throughout the year, so choosing the right time for your visit is essential. Generally, the most favourable time to travel is during the cool, dry season. Typically lasts from November to February.

In the north, including Luang Prabang and Vientiane, the climate is characterised by three seasons: a cool, dry period from November to February, a hot season from March to May, and a rainy season from June to October. Therefore, the ideal time to explore this region is between November and February, when the weather is cooler and more comfortable.

Central and southern Laos, encompassing cities like Pakse and the 4,000 Islands region, experiences a tropical monsoon climate. The hot season occurs from March to May, followed by the rainy season from June to October, and the cool, dry season from November to February. Therefore, the most favourable time to visit this area is during the cool season when the temperatures are more pleasant, and the humidity is lower.

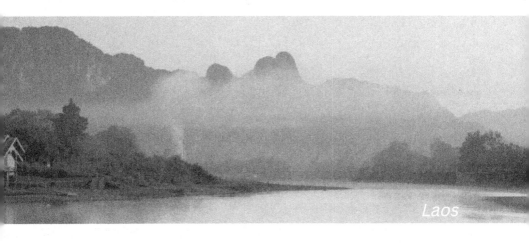

Laos

Cambodia

The climate in Cambodia varies throughout the year, making it crucial to select the appropriate time for your visit. Generally, the most favourable time to travel is during the cool, dry season, which usually extends from November to February.

Cambodia experiences a tropical monsoon climate with two primary seasons: the wet season, from May to October, and the dry season, lasting from November to April. The dry season can be further divided into the cool dry period from November to February and the dry period from March to April.

The cool, dry period is ideal for exploring Cambodia, including popular destinations like Phnom Penh, Siem Reap, and the Angkor Wat temple complex. In addition, the weather is cooler and more comfortable during this time, making it perfect for sightseeing and outdoor activities. The hot, dry period from March to April can be sweltering, often reaching 40°C (104°F).

The wet season brings heavy rain, particularly from July to September. While the rain may cause travel disruptions, it transforms the countryside into a lush, green landscape. Travelling during this season is possible, but be prepared for occasional downpours and slippery conditions.

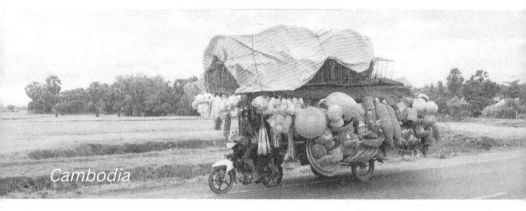

Cambodia

Vietnam

In the north, including Hanoi, the climate is characterised by a distinct winter and summer, with a cool, dry winter lasting from November to April and a hot, humid summer from May to October.

Central Vietnam, encompassing cities like Hue, Da Nang, and Hoi An, experiences a hot and dry climate from January to August, with occasional typhoons from September to November.

In the south, including Ho Chi Minh City and the Mekong Delta, the climate is tropical with high humidity. The dry season lasts from December to April, while the wet season occurs from May to November. The most favourable time to explore this region is during the dry season, particularly from December to February when temperatures are relatively cooler and more comfortable.

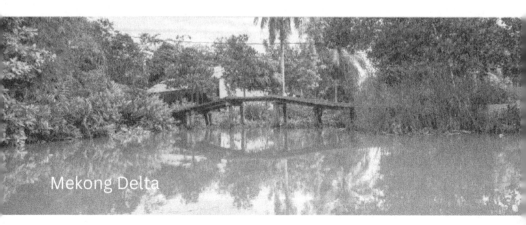

Mekong Delta

NOTES

CHAPTER 11
To See or Do

Southeast Asia is a diverse and vibrant region with a rich history, fascinating cultures, and stunning natural landscapes. There is indeed plenty to see and do for travellers. Here are some top attractions for each country:

Thailand

Explore the Grand Palace: The Grand Palace in Bangkok is an architectural marvel and the former residence of Thai kings. Visit the Temple of the Emerald Buddha (Wat Phra Kaew), situated within the palace grounds, which houses a Buddha statue carved from a single jade stone.

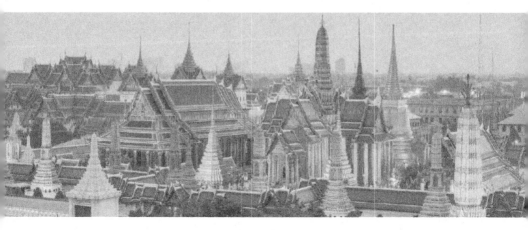

Discover ancient Ayutthaya: Once the capital of the Kingdom of Siam, Ayutthaya is now a UNESCO World Heritage Site, featuring impressive temples, palaces, and ruins. Spend a day exploring the historical wonders of this ancient city.

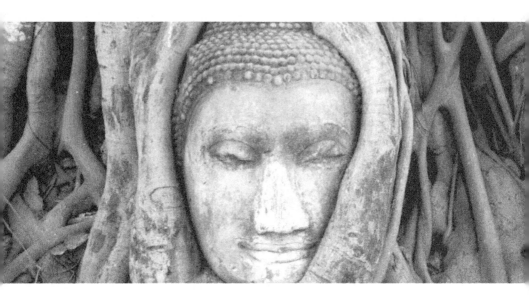

Exploring Chiang Mai: Nestled in the mountains of northern Thailand, Chiang Mai offers a more relaxed atmosphere than bustling Bangkok. Explore its numerous temples, including the famous Wat Phra That Doi Suthep, and visit the vibrant night markets.

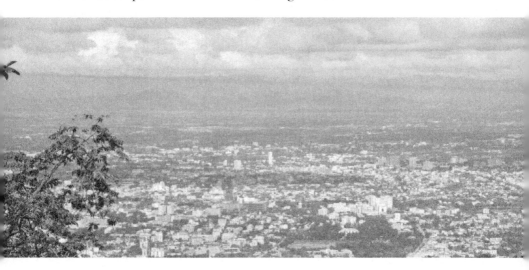

<u>Unwind on idyllic islands:</u> Thailand is home to some of the world's most beautiful islands, such as Phuket, Koh Samui, and Koh Phi Phi. Enjoy pristine beaches, crystal-clear waters, and fantastic snorkelling or diving experiences.

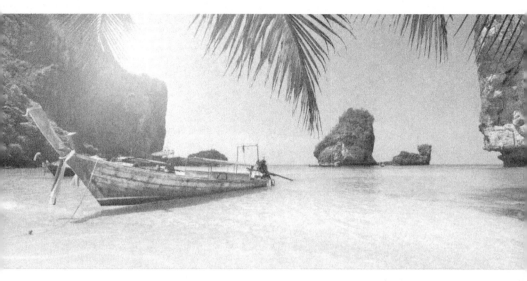

<u>Experience Thai cuisine:</u> Sample the incredible flavours of Thai food, from delicious street food to fine dining. Don't miss dishes like pad Thai, green curry, and mango sticky rice.

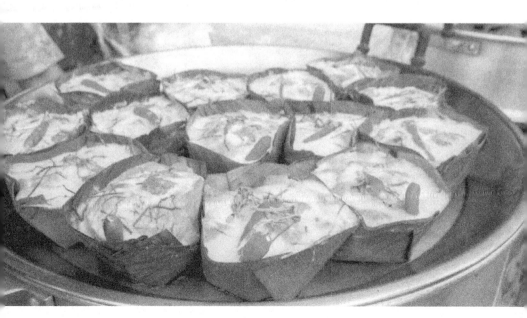

Witness Thai festival: Plan your trip around one of Thailand's many festivals, such as Songkran (Thai New Year) or Loy Krathong (Festival of Lights), to experience the rich culture and traditions of the country.

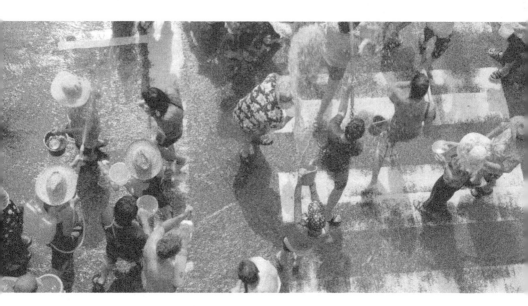

Explore the vibrant city of Bangkok: Immerse yourself in the bustling streets of Bangkok, where you can visit iconic sites like Wat Arun, the Temple of Dawn, and the bustling Chatuchak Weekend Market.

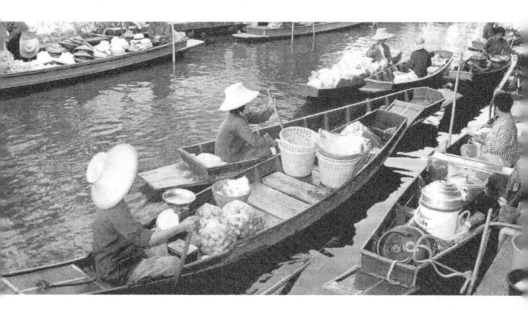

Connect with nature in Khao Sok National Park: This stunning national park in southern Thailand offers a lush, unspoiled environment for trekking, wildlife spotting, and exploring the mesmerising Cheow Lan Lake.

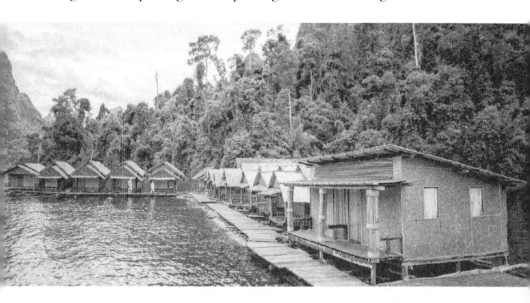

Visit the historic town of Sukhothai: Another UNESCO World Heritage Site, Sukhothai was the first capital of Siam. Wander through the well-preserved ruins and appreciate the early Siamese architecture.

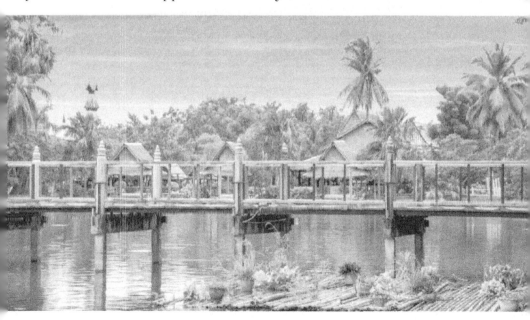

Laos

Explore Luang Prabang: This charming UNESCO World Heritage town is brimming with history, culture, and beautiful French colonial architecture. Visit the numerous temples, such as Wat Xieng Thong, and wander the night markets for local handicrafts and street food.

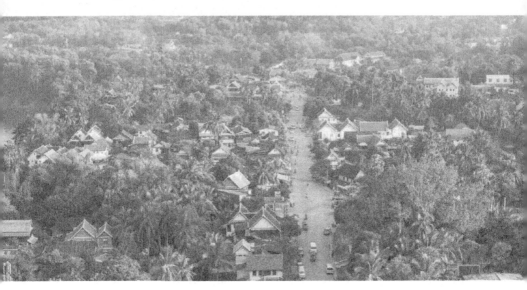

Discover the ancient city of Vientiane: The capital city of Laos offers a wealth of cultural sites, including the stunning golden stupa of Pha That Luang, the national symbol of Laos, and the Patuxai Victory Monument, reminiscent of the Arc de Triomphe.

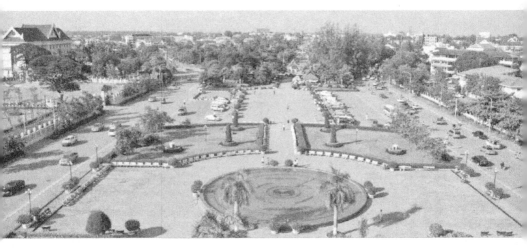

To See Or Do

<u>Visit the Plain of Jars:</u> One of Laos's most mysterious archaeological sites, the Plain of Jars features thousands of large stone jars scattered across the landscape, providing a fascinating insight into the region's ancient history.

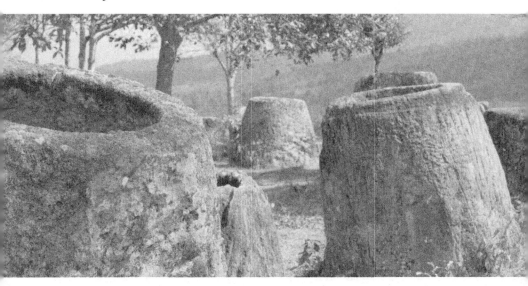

<u>Admire the natural beauty of the Kuang Si Waterfalls:</u> Located near Luang Prabang, these picturesque waterfalls offer a perfect opportunity for swimming, hiking, or simply enjoying the breathtaking scenery.

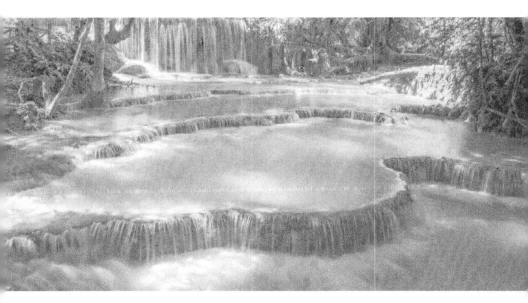

<u>Cruise along the Mekong River:</u> Experience the serene beauty of Laos by taking a boat trip along the Mekong River, which offers stunning views of the lush countryside, traditional villages, and abundant wildlife.

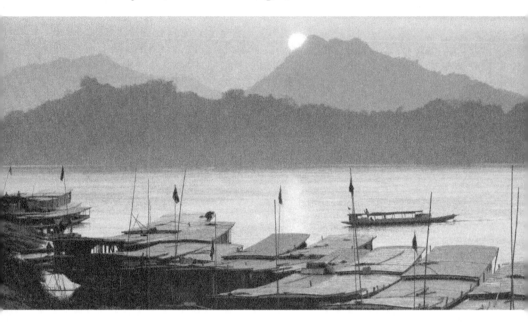

<u>The Bolaven Plateau:</u> This elevated region in southern Laos is home to verdant forests, spectacular waterfalls, and fertile land ideal for growing coffee and tea. Take a guided tour to sample local produce and admire the stunning landscapes.

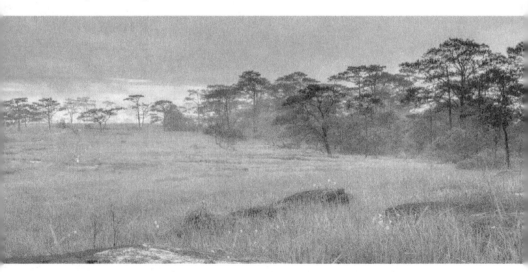

Explore the 4,000 Islands (Si Phan Don): This picturesque region in the Mekong River is home to numerous islands, waterfalls, and traditional villages. Cycle the islands, or take a boat trip to spot the rare Irrawaddy dolphins. There are said to be less than 100 Irrawaddy dolphins.

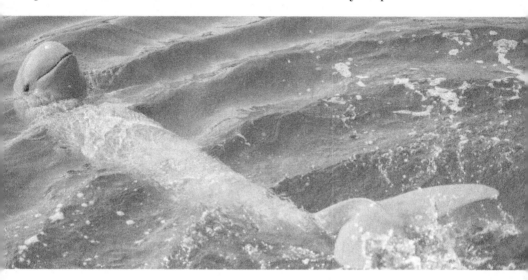

Visit Wat Phu: This ancient Khmer temple complex is a UNESCO World Heritage Site and offers a fascinating glimpse into Laos's history. Wander through the well-preserved ruins, admiring the intricate carvings and stunning views of the surrounding countryside.

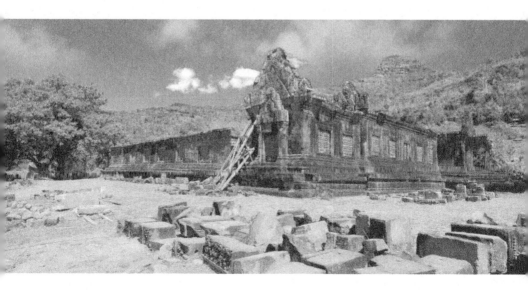

<u>Experience delicious Laotian cuisine:</u> Savour the unique flavours of Laotian food, which includes dishes like sticky rice, laap (minced meat salad), and tam mak hoong (spicy green papaya salad).

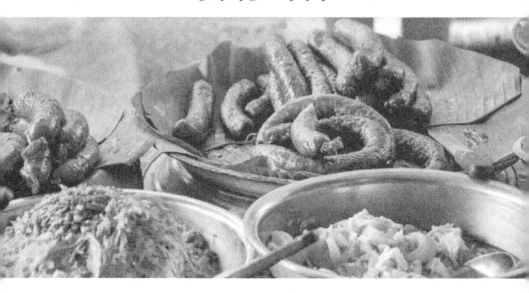

<u>Immerse yourself in local culture:</u> Participate in a traditional Baci ceremony, a significant Laotian ritual to celebrate special occasions or welcome visitors. The ceremony involves tying symbolic threads around participants' wrists to bring good luck and harmony.

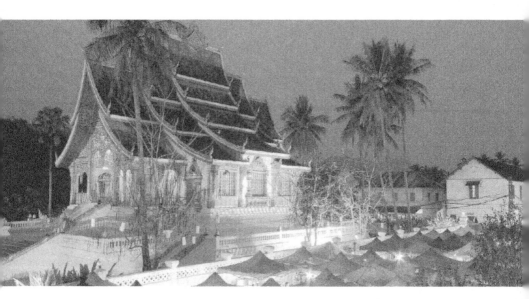

Cambodia

<u>Visit Angkor Wat:</u> Angkor Wat is a temple complex in Cambodia near the modern city of Siem Reap. It is the largest religious monument in the world. Cycling through this incredible site is not to be missed.

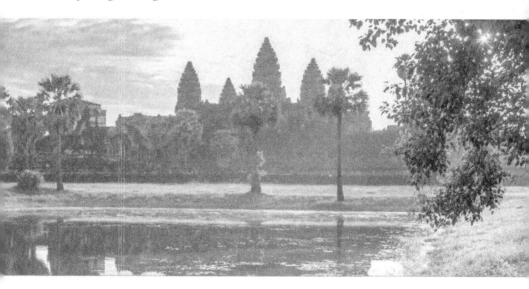

<u>Tour the Killing Fields of Choeung Ek:</u> This is a mass grave site and memorial located about 15km (9m) south of Phnom Penh, Cambodia. It is a haunting reminder of the atrocities committed by the Khmer Rouge regime, led by Pol Pot, between 1975 and 1979.

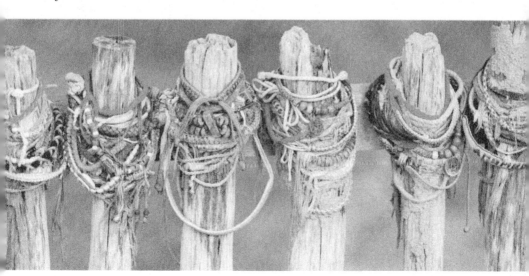

The Royal Palace in Phnom Penh: It is the official residence of the King of Cambodia and a symbol of the country's monarchy. It is an exquisite example of traditional Khmer architecture and an important cultural and historical landmark.

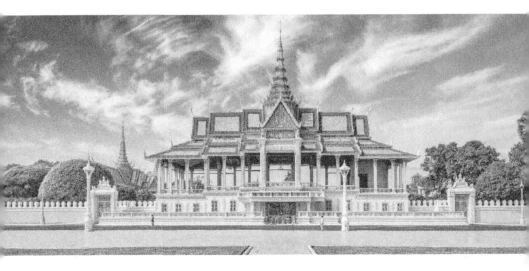

Take a boat tour of Tonle Sap Lake: Tonle Sap Lake is the largest freshwater lake in Southeast Asia, located in the heart of Cambodia. It plays a vital role in the country's ecology, economy, and culture. The lake is unique for its size, biodiversity, and significant seasonal variations in its water levels.

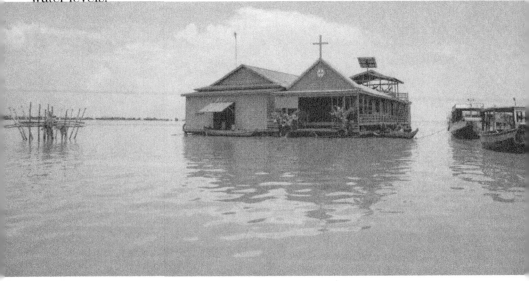

Koh Rong: Koh Rong Island is a tropical paradise off the coast of Sihanoukville, Cambodia. Known for its pristine white-sand beaches, crystal-clear turquoise waters, and lush jungle interior, the island offers visitors an idyllic setting to relax, unwind, and enjoy various outdoor activities.

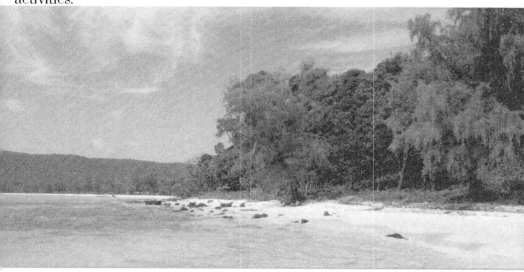

Phnom Penh Night Market: Experience the vibrant nightlife and sample local street food at this bustling market. It is a popular destination for locals and tourists to indulge in delicious Cambodian street food.

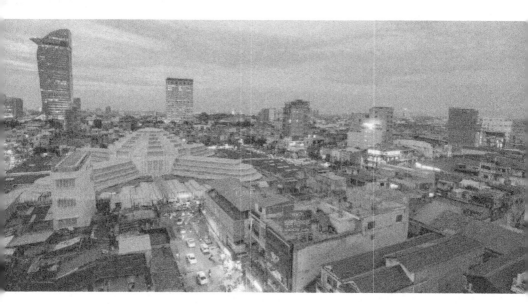

Bokor Hill Station: Bokor Hill Station, located in Preah Monivong Bokor National Park in southern Cambodia, is an abandoned French colonial hill station and a popular day trip destination for those seeking to explore its mysterious ruins and enjoy stunning panoramic views.

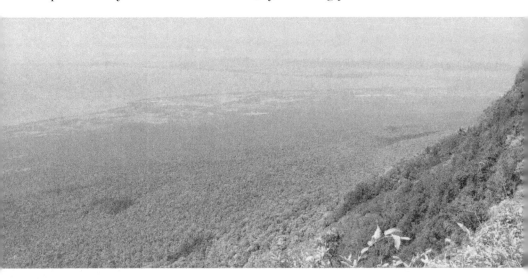

The Silver Pagoda: The Silver Pagoda, also known as Wat Preah Keo Morokat or the Temple of the Emerald Buddha, is a stunning pagoda within the Royal Palace complex in Phnom Penh, Cambodia. It is an important religious and cultural site, housing many precious treasures and artefacts.

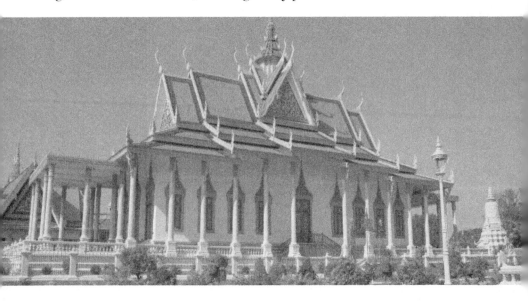

Preah Vihear Temple: Trek through the jungle to this remote and breathtaking temple on the Cambodian-Thai border. Preah Vihear Temple is an ancient Hindu temple dedicated to Lord Shiva, located on a cliff in the Dângrêk Mountains, near the border between Cambodia and Thailand.

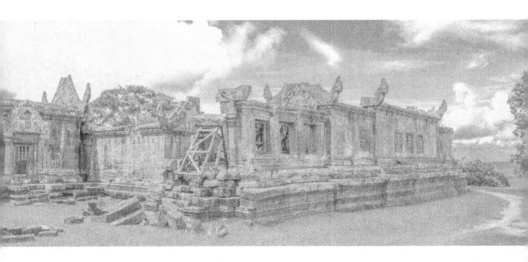

Battambang Bamboo Train: Ride the unique bamboo train through rural Cambodia and enjoy the beautiful countryside scenery. The Bamboo Train is a simple, improvised rail vehicle consisting of a flat bamboo platform mounted on two wheels powered by a small gasoline engine. It runs on a single track and can reach up to 40 km/h (25 mph) speeds.

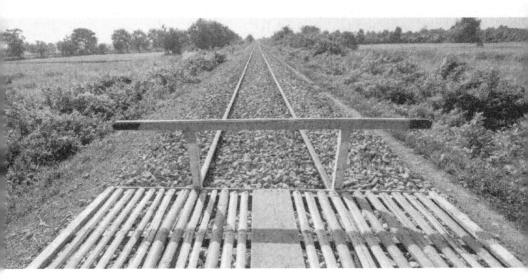

Vietnam

 Visit Vietnam's largest island: Phu Quoc is the largest island in Vietnam, located in the Gulf of Thailand off the southern coast of the country, near the border with Cambodia. The island is part of the Kien Giang province and covers an area of 574 square kilometers (222 square miles).

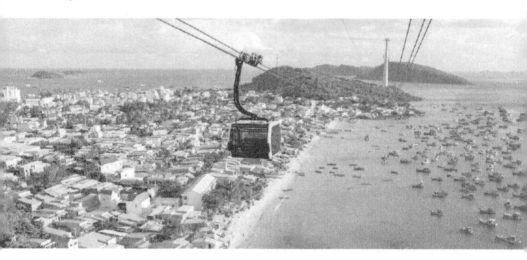

Ha Long Bay: Take a boat tour through this stunning UNESCO World Heritage site with its towering limestone cliffs and turquoise waters.

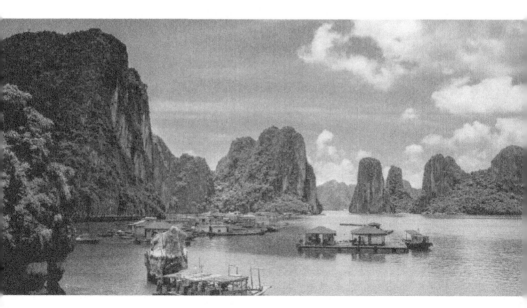

Cu Chi Tunnels: The Cu Chi Tunnels are an extensive network of underground tunnels located about 40km (25m) northwest of Ho Chi Minh City (formerly Saigon) in Vietnam. The tunnels were originally dug by the Viet Minh during the First Indochina War against the French in the late 1940s and expanded by the Viet Cong during the Vietnam War

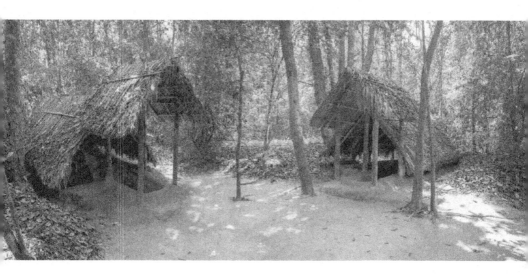

Ho Chi Minh City: Visit this bustling metropolis with its impressive colonial architecture, lively markets, and delicious street food.

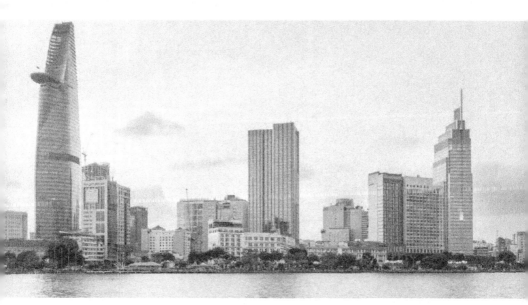

Phong Nha-Ke Bang National Park: Phong Nha-Ke Bang National Park is a UNESCO World Heritage Site in the Quang Binh province of north-central Vietnam. The park is renowned for its stunning limestone karst formations, vast caves and grottoes, pristine jungle, and diverse flora and fauna.

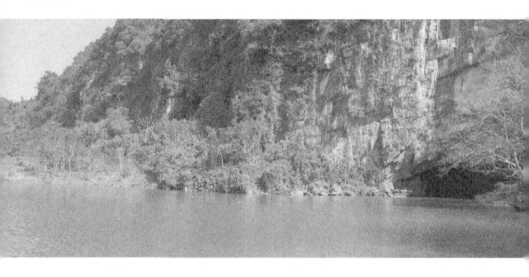

Sapa: Trek through this beautiful region's stunning rice terraces and mountains and experience the traditional way of life of the ethnic minority communities.

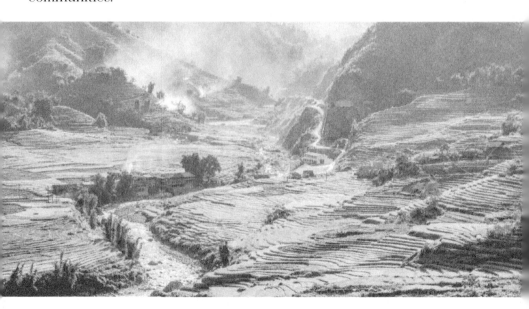

<u>Hue:</u> Hue is a historical city in central Vietnam, approximately midway between Hanoi and Ho Chi Minh City. It was the capital of the Nguyen Dynasty, which ruled Vietnam from 1802 until 1945, and the seat of the imperial court.

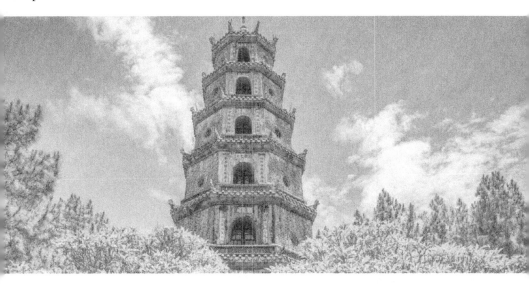

<u>Hoi An:</u> Hoi An is a well-preserved ancient town in Quang Nam Province on the central coast of Vietnam. Recognized as a UNESCO World Heritage Site since 1999, Hoi An is famous for its rich history, cultural heritage, and unique blend of architectural styles,

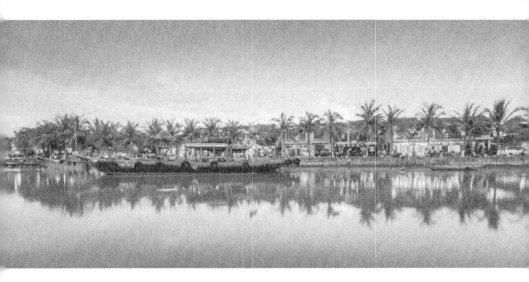

Ninh Binh: Visit this beautiful region with its stunning karst mountains, tranquil rivers, and ancient temples, often called the "Halong Bay on Land".

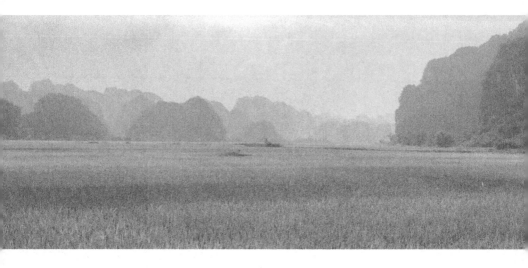

Mekong Delta: Take a boat tour of this lush and fertile region, known as the "rice bowl" of Vietnam, and witness the traditional way of life of the river communities.

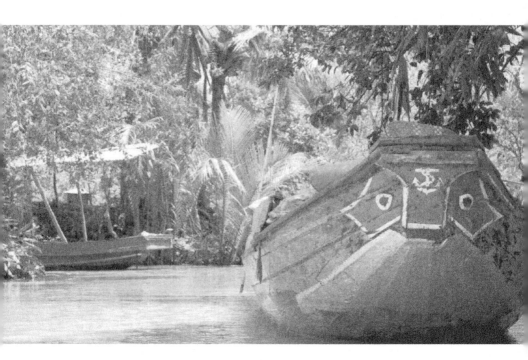

CHAPTER 12
Wildlife Dangers

Southeast Asia is celebrated for its abundant biodiversity, verdant landscapes, and enchanting flora and fauna. Nevertheless, visitors must be aware of the potential dangers of certain poisonous and perilous plants and animals amidst this natural magnificence. In this article, we shall delve into some of the most hazardous species found in the region. In addition, we will provide images of this remarkable wildlife wherever possible. But, as you undoubtedly do, we also recognise that most creatures and plants are unlikely to pose a threat unless disturbed or encountered by chance. As for plants, knowing what not to put in contact with delicate skin can be helpful, given the nature of cycle tourists and budget travellers.

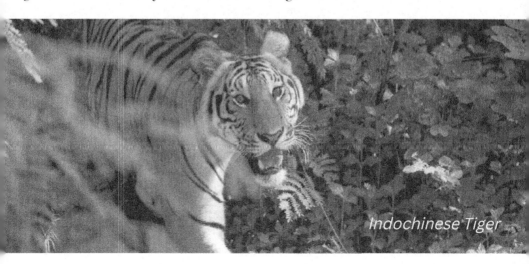

Indochinese Tiger

Plants

Southeast Asia is celebrated for its diverse and abundant flora. It is home to an estimated 15,000 vascular plant species, many displaying vibrant colours and unique shapes. However, several dangerous plants are hidden amidst this botanical paradise, posing risks to human and animal health. This article explores many potentially harmful plants native to the region, which might not look so harmful.

Dendrocnide meyeniana (Stinging Tree): A notorious plant in Thailand is the Dendrocnide meyeniana, commonly known as the stinging tree or Gympie-Gympie in Australia. This large shrub or small tree is native to Southeast Asia and is covered in tiny, hair-like structures called trichomes. These trichomes contain a potent neurotoxin that causes excruciating pain when they come into contact with the skin. The pain has been described as similar to being burned with hot acid or electrocuted and can persist for days or even weeks. If you suspect you have come into contact with the tree, seek medical attention promptly.

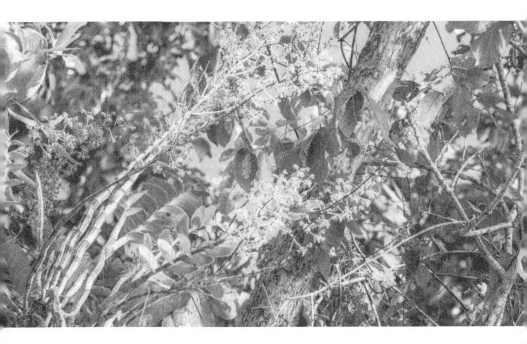

<u>Alocasia macrorrhizos (Giant Taro)</u>: The Alocasia macrorrhizos, or giant taro, is a large, tropical plant. Although cultivated for its edible tubers, the plant contains calcium oxalate crystals, which can cause irritation and burning sensations if ingested or touched. Eating large quantities of giant taro can lead to severe symptoms such as vomiting, diarrhoea, and difficulty breathing. To avoid accidental contact with the plant, wear protective gloves when handling or consuming giant taro, and ensure it is thoroughly cooked before consumption.

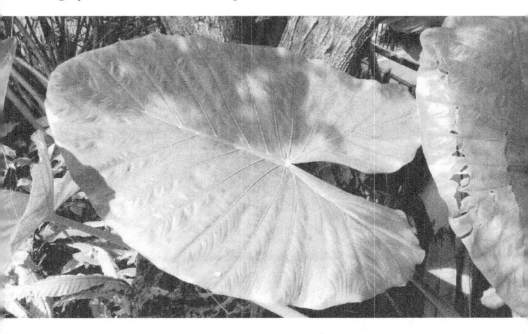

<u>Dieffenbachia seguine (Dumb Cane)</u>: Dieffenbachia seguine, also known as dumb cane, is a popular ornamental plant. This attractive plant, however, hides a toxic secret. Its sap contains calcium oxalate crystals, which can cause a range of symptoms if ingested, such as the mouth and throat irritation, drooling, difficulty swallowing, and even temporary speech loss, hence the name "dumb cane." In severe cases, ingestion can lead to difficulty breathing, vomiting, and diarrhoea. To prevent exposure to dumb cane, keep the plant out of reach of children and pets and wear gloves when handling or pruning the plant.

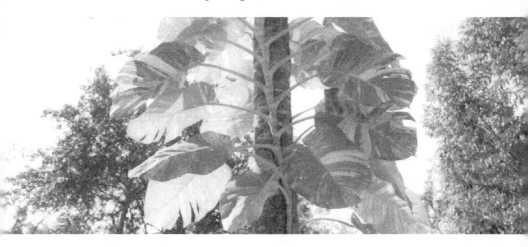

Ricinus communis (Castor Bean): The castor bean plant is native to the Mediterranean, Eastern Africa, and India but has become naturalised in Southeast Asia. While castor oil, derived from the plant's seeds, has numerous medicinal and industrial uses, they are highly toxic. They contain ricin, a potent toxin that can cause severe symptoms if ingested, such as nausea, vomiting, abdominal pain, and internal bleeding. Ingestion of even a small number of seeds can be fatal. Avoid handling or consuming castor beans and keep the plant away from children and pets.

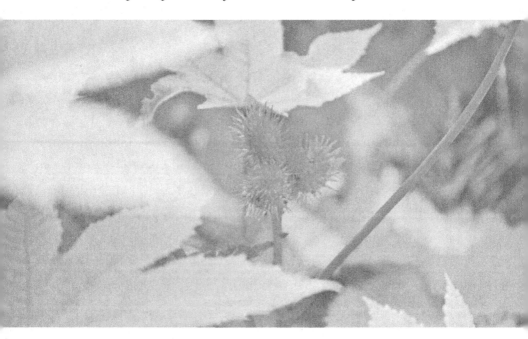

Jatropha curcas (Physic Nut): Jatropha curcas, or physic nut, is a small tree or large shrub native to Central and South America but has been introduced to Southeast Asia as a source of biodiesel. While the oil extracted from the seeds has various applications, they are highly toxic. Ingestion can lead to severe gastrointestinal symptoms, such as nausea, vomiting, abdominal pain, dehydration, dizziness, and weakness.

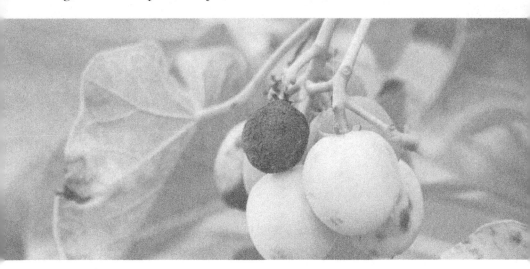

Suicide Tree (Cerbera odollam): This tree bears fruits resembling small mangoes, but the seeds contain a potent toxin called cerberin, which can be fatal if ingested. Avoid consuming any part of this plant and educate children about its dangers.

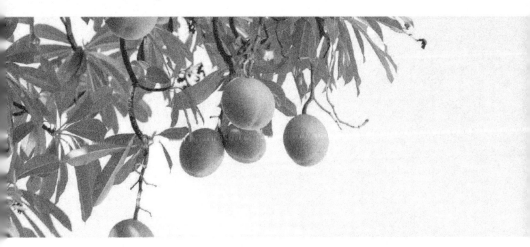

Flame Lily (Gloriosa superba): All parts of the flame lily are toxic, containing colchicine, which can cause gastrointestinal distress, kidney failure, and even death if ingested. Avoid handling or consuming any part of this plant.

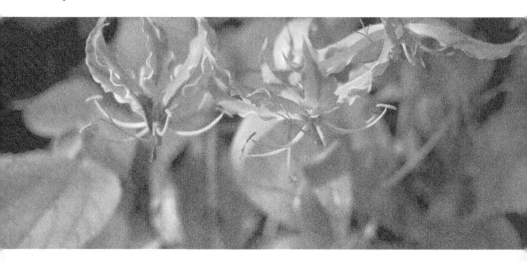

Yellow Oleander (Thevetia peruviana): The yellow oleander is an attractive ornamental plant, but all parts are poisonous, containing cardiac glycosides that can affect the heart. Ingestion can cause nausea, vomiting, dizziness, and potentially fatal cardiac complications.

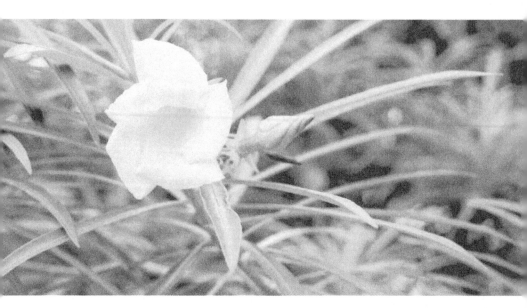

Sea Creatures

If you're considering a refreshing plunge to escape the sweltering heat and humidity, it's essential to be mindful of some specific hazards that may be present.

Box Jellyfish (Chironex fleckeri): Box jellyfish are dangerous. While uncommon, encounters with these venomous creatures can result in painful and sometimes life-threatening stings.

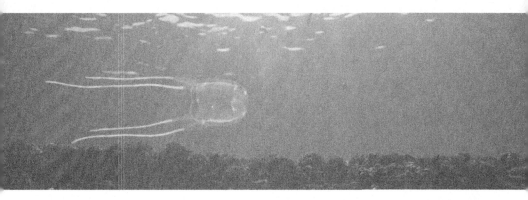

Stonefish (Synanceia spp): The stonefish is a highly venomous marine creature. They are known for their excellent camouflage, allowing them to blend seamlessly with their rocky or coral surroundings.

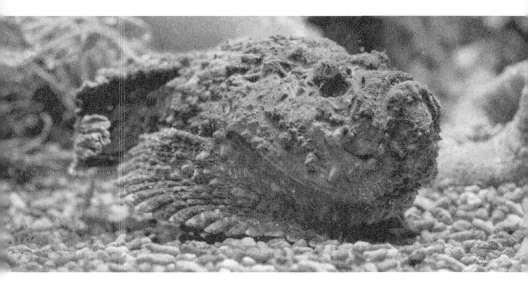

Banded Sea Krait (Laticauda semifasciata): Sea snakes are generally not aggressive and tend to avoid humans. However, they may bite if they feel threatened or cornered.

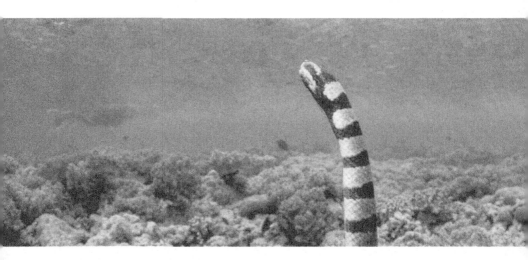

Portuguese Man o' War (Physalia physalis): is a marine creature known for its venomous tentacles, which can deliver painful and sometimes dangerous stings. They are primarily found in the Atlantic Ocean but have been occasionally reported in the waters of Southeast Asia, particularly during certain seasons or when ocean currents carry them to the region.

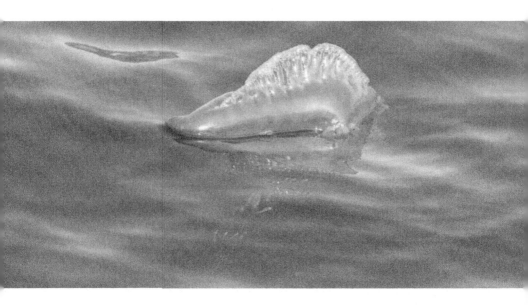

Insects And Other Bugs

Southeast Asia is home to various insects and bugs, some of which can pose risks to humans. While most insects in the region are harmless, it's essential to be aware of those that can cause harm.

Mosquitoes (Aedes, Anopheles, and Culex species): Mosquitoes are notorious for transmitting diseases such as dengue fever, malaria, and chikungunya. Use insect repellent, wear long-sleeved clothing, and sleep under a mosquito net or in an air-conditioned room.

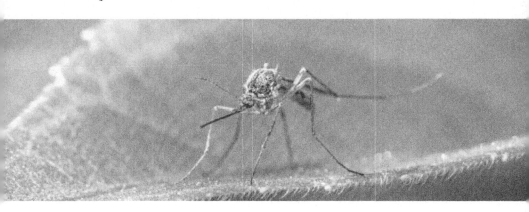

Scorpions (Heterometrus laoticus and other species): Southeast Asia is home to several species of scorpions, some of which possess venom capable of causing severe pain, swelling, and in rare cases, anaphylaxis. To avoid scorpion encounters, be cautious when lifting rocks or logs and always shake out shoes and clothing before wearing them.

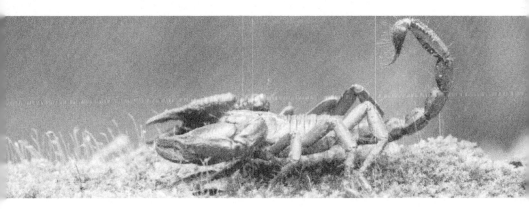

Centipedes (Scolopendra species): Giant centipedes can grow up to 30 centimetres long and are equipped with venomous fangs that can inflict painful bites. While centipede bites are rarely life-threatening, they can cause extreme pain, swelling, and sometimes, fever or dizziness. Exercise caution when exploring rocky or forested areas and avoid handling.

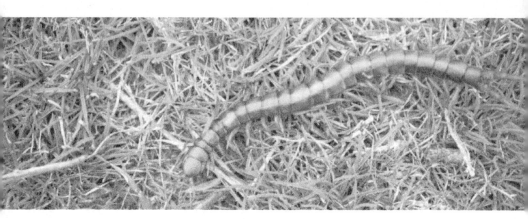

Black Widow Spider (Latrodectus hasselti): The Black Widow Spider, known for its distinctive red hourglass marking on its abdomen, can deliver a potent neurotoxic venom. Bites from this spider can cause muscle pain, nausea, and difficulty breathing and may require medical attention.

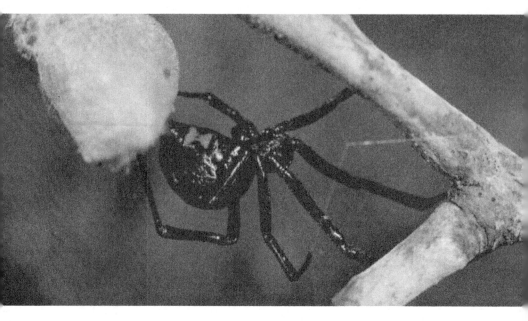

<u>Brown Recluse Spider (Loxosceles reclusa)</u>: The brown recluse has a venomous bite which can require medical attention but rarely fatal.

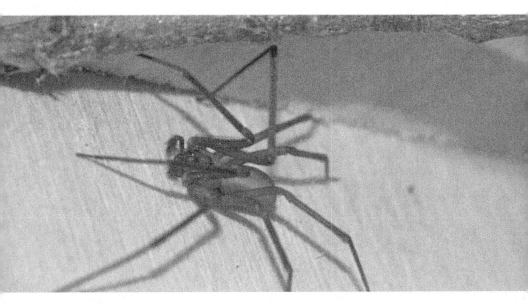

Snakes

Southeast Asia has more than 200 species, of which approximately 60 are venomous.

<u>King Cobra (Ophiophagus hannah)</u>: The King Cobra is the world's longest venomous snake, capable of growing up to 5.5 metres. Although generally shy and elusive, it is highly venomous and should be cautiously treated.

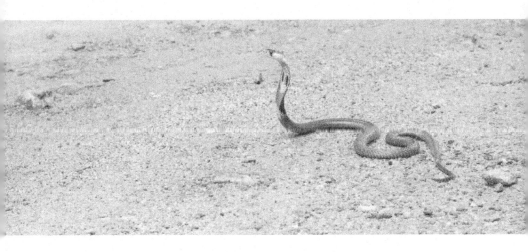

<u>Banded Krait (Bungarus fasciatus):</u> The Banded Krait is easily identified by its alternating black and yellow bands. Its venom is highly potent, containing neurotoxins and myotoxins, which can cause muscle paralysis and respiratory failure.

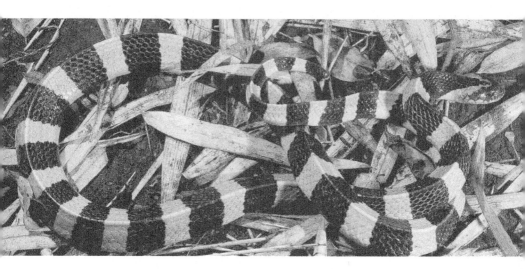

Thailand is home to several species of venomous snakes, including several species of vipers. Here are some of the vipers you might encounter in Thailand: Malayan Pit Viper, Wagler's Pit Viper, Russell's Viper, Pope's Pit Viper, Siamese Peninsula Pit Viper.

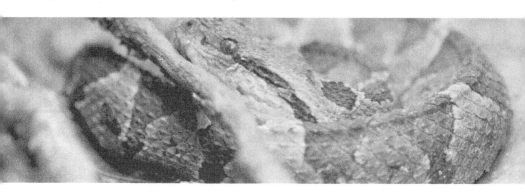

If you encounter a snake in Southeast Asia, it's essential to exercise caution and avoid approaching or handling it. If you're bitten, seek medical attention immediately.

Larger Land Animals

Southeast Asia is home to various large land animals, some of which can be potentially dangerous if encountered in the wild. The chances of experiencing these animals in the wild are low, and they generally avoid human contact. Some of the potentially dangerous large animals include:

Elephants: The Asian elephant (Elephas maximus) is native to Southeast Asia and is the region's largest land mammal. While they are usually gentle and docile, they can be dangerous when threatened or provoked. The estimated maximum population: Thailand, Laos, Cambodia, Vietnam: 4650

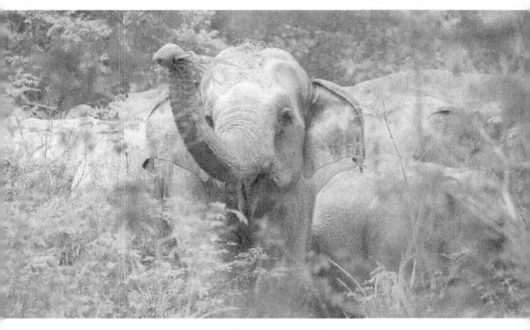

Tigers: The Indochinese tiger (Panthera tigris corbetti) and Malayan tiger (Panthera tigris jacksoni) are native to parts of Southeast Asia. Although tiger populations have declined significantly due to habitat loss and poaching, they can pose a risk if encountered in the wild. The estimated maximum population: Thailand, Laos, Cambodia, Vietnam: 227.

It's worth noting that these estimates are just that - estimates.

<u>Wild Boars:</u> In Southeast Asia, wild boars (Sus scrofa) are generally shy and avoid humans. However, they can become aggressive if threatened, particularly when protecting their young. The estimated maximum population: Thailand, Laos, Cambodia, Vietnam: 7.2m.

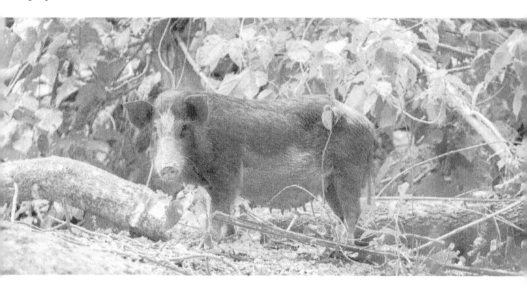

<u>Leopards:</u> Indochinese leopard (Panthera pardus delacouri), a subspecies of the leopard (Panthera pardus). They inhabit various types of forests, including tropical rainforests, deciduous forests, and evergreen forests. The estimated maximum population: Thailand, Laos, Cambodia, Vietnam: 950.

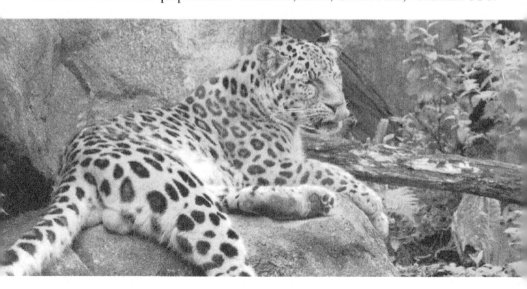

Asiatic Black Bear: Also known as the moon bear, is easily distinguishable by the white or cream-coloured V-shaped mark on its chest, with males weighing 100-200 kg and females weighing 65-125 kg. The IUCN estimates that there are likely fewer than 10,000 moon bears left in Southeast Asia.

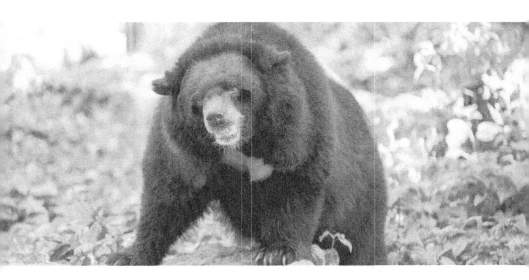

Sun Bear: The sun bear is the smallest of all bear species, with adult males weighing between 30-70 kg and females weighing between 20-40 kg. Its name is derived from the golden or white crescent-shaped marking on its chest, which resembles a rising sun. The IUCN estimates that there are likely fewer than 10,000 sun bears left in the wild in Southeast Asia

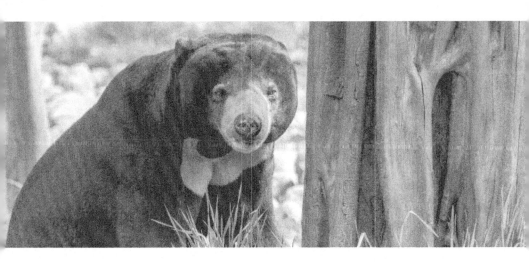

<u>Wild buffalo:</u> Though the wild buffalo population is stable, they are an uncommon sight in Southeast Asia, primarily found in protected areas or remote regions. The wild buffalo, also known as the Asian water buffalo or the wild Asian buffalo, is a separate species from the domesticated water buffalo but closely related.

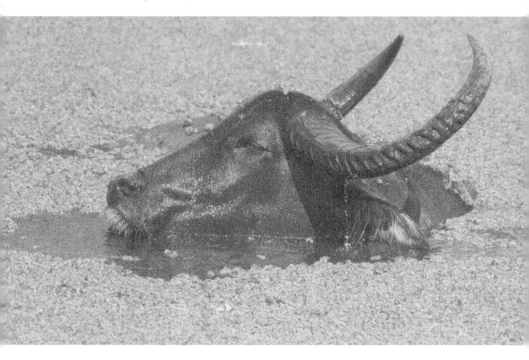

Whilst Southeast Asia is home to diverse wildlife, some species can threaten human safety. Therefore, both locals and visitors must exercise caution and remain vigilant of potential dangers when venturing into the natural habitats of these animals. Although the overall risks to health are low, this region's unique flora and fauna offer spectacular sights worth cherishing and appreciating.

CHAPTER 13
A Brief History Of Thailand

Population (2023):	70 Million+
Leading religion:	Buddhism
Currency:	Thai Baht
Politics and stature:	Constitutional monarchy
National sport:	Muay Thai
Average age:	39
Urbanization:	52 percent
National dish:	Pad Thai
National animal:	Elephant
National plant/flower:	Cassia Fistula Linn

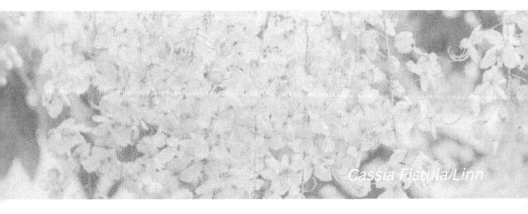

Cassia Fistula Linn

Introduction

Thailand, known as the Land of Smiles, is a Southeast Asian country with a rich and colourful history. From its early days as a collection of small kingdoms to its current status as a constitutional monarchy, Thailand has experienced many cultural, political, and social changes throughout the centuries. This brief history will provide an overview of the key events and developments that have shaped today's nation.

Early Kingdoms and Civilisations (1st to 13th century)

The history of Thailand can be traced back to prehistoric times, with archaeological evidence suggesting human habitation in the region for at least 40,000 years. The first recorded civilisations in what is now Thailand emerged around the 1st century AD, notably the Mon and Khmer cultures.

The Mon people established the Dvaravati Kingdom in present-day central Thailand. They were heavily influenced by Indian culture, and the kingdom flourished as a centre of trade and Buddhism from the 6th to the 11th century.

Meanwhile, the Khmer Empire, centred in modern-day Cambodia, expanded its influence across the region, including parts of Thailand. The Khmer built impressive temples and cities, such as the famous Angkor Wat, which still stands today as a testament to their architectural prowess.

The Birth of Thai Kingdoms (13th to 14th century)

The early 13th century marked the emergence of the Thai kingdom, the Sukhothai Kingdom, founded by King Sri Indraditya. This period is often regarded as the 'golden age' of Thai history, with significant developments in art, culture, and politics. King Ramkhamhaeng, the third ruler of Sukhothai, is credited with the creation of the Thai script, which is still used today.

Towards the end of the 13th century, another Thai kingdom, the Lanna Kingdom, emerged in northern Thailand. Founded by King Mengrai, it was centred around Chiang Mai. The Lanna Kingdom flourished for several centuries, cultivating a distinctive culture and language.

The Ayutthaya Period (1351-1767)

The Ayutthaya Kingdom, founded by King U Thong (Ramathibodi I) in 1351, rose to prominence as the dominant power in the region. Ayutthaya, the kingdom's capital, was located on an island at the confluence of three rivers and grew to become one of the world's largest and most cosmopolitan cities at the time.

For over 400 years, the Ayutthaya Kingdom experienced growth and prosperity thanks to its strategic location for trade and diplomacy. However, it faced numerous challenges, including internal power struggles and conflicts with neighbouring kingdoms, such as the Burmese and the Khmer.

The kingdom ended in 1767 when the Burmese invaded and sacked Ayutthaya. The city was destroyed, and many historical records and artefacts were lost, marking the end of a significant chapter in Thai history.

The Thonburi and Rattanakosin Periods (1767-1932)

Following the fall of Ayutthaya, General Taksin emerged as a national hero and established a new capital in Thonburi across the Chao Phraya River from present-day Bangkok. Taksin reunited the shattered kingdom and repelled further Burmese invasions. However, his reign was short-lived, and he was overthrown in a coup in 1782.

The coup leader, General Chao Phraya Chakri, then founded the Rattanakosin Kingdom and established Bangkok as the new capital. He became King Rama I, the first monarch of the Chakri Dynasty, which continues to reign in Thailand to this day.

During the Rattanakosin period, the kingdom expanded its territory and influence, incorporating neighbouring regions such as Lanna and parts of Laos, Cambodia, and Malaysia.

In the 19th century, under the reigns of King Rama IV (Mongkut) and King Rama V (Chulalongkorn), Thailand experienced significant modernisation and reform. These monarchs embraced Western ideas and technology, introduced educational and legal reforms, and established diplomatic relations with European powers. Notably, Thailand (then known as Siam) managed to maintain its independence throughout the colonial era, making it the only country in Southeast Asia to avoid European colonisation.

The 1932 Revolution and the Transition to a Constitutional Monarchy

On 24 June 1932, a bloodless coup led by a group of military officers and civil servants, known as the People's Party (Khana Ratsadon), overthrew the absolute monarchy. King Rama VII (Prajadhipok) agreed to establish a constitutional monarchy, and the first constitution was promulgated on 10 December 1932, now celebrated as Thailand's Constitution Day.

However, the transition to a constitutional monarchy could have been smoother. Instead, the following decades witnessed political instability, with numerous coups, constitutional changes, and short-lived governments. In addition, the involvement of military factions and the rise of communist movements in the region further complicated Thailand's political landscape.

World War II and the Cold War Era

During World War II, Thailand declared neutrality but was later forced to allow Japanese troops to pass through its territory. In 1941, Thailand signed an alliance with Japan, and in 1942, it declared war on the United States and the United Kingdom. After the war, Thailand became a US ally, receiving economic and military aid to counter the spread of communism.

Throughout the Cold War, Thailand played a strategic role in the region, hosting US military bases and supporting anti-communist efforts in neighbouring countries, such as Vietnam and Laos. The country also experienced rapid economic growth, transforming itself from an agrarian society to an industrialised nation.

Modern Thailand (1980s to the present)

Since the 1980s, Thailand has undergone significant political, economic, and social changes. The country has become more democratic, with increased political participation and the emergence of a vibrant civil society. However, political instability and military coups have persisted, notably in 2006 and 2014.

Thailand's economy has continued to grow, becoming a regional leader in the tourism, manufacturing, and technology sectors. The nation has also experienced challenges like income inequality, environmental degradation, and human rights issues.

Throughout its history, Thailand has maintained a unique and distinct cultural identity, marked by a deep reverence for the monarchy, the prevalence of Buddhism, and a strong sense of national pride. As the country continues to evolve and adapt to the challenges of the modern world, it remains firmly rooted in its rich historical and cultural heritage.

CHAPTER 14

A Brief History Of Laos

Population (2023):	7.5 Million+
Leading religion:	Buddhism
Currency:	Laotian Kip
Politics and stature:	Socialist republic with a single-party communist government
National sport:	Muay Lao
Average age:	22
Urbanization:	52 percent
National dish:	Larb
National animal:	Elephant
National plant:	Dok Champa

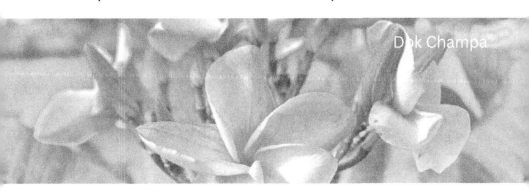

Dok Champa

Introduction

Laos, officially the Laotian People's Democratic Republic, is a landlocked country in Southeast Asia, bordered by China, Vietnam, Cambodia, Thailand, and Myanmar. Its history is marked by its strategic location, complex relationship with its neighbours, and rich cultural heritage. This brief history will offer an overview of the key events and developments that have shaped the nation we know today.

Early Civilisations and Kingdoms (1st to 14th century)

The early history of Laos is intertwined with the story of the broader Southeast Asian region. Archaeological evidence suggests that the area now known as Laos was inhabited as early as 10,000 years ago. The first notable civilisation in the region was the Indianised kingdom of Funan, which emerged in the 1st century AD and spanned across parts of present-day Laos, Vietnam, and Cambodia.

Between the 6th and 8th centuries, the Mon and Khmer kingdoms, influenced by Indian culture, Buddhism, and Hinduism, established their presence in the region. They created impressive temples and cities, some of which are cultural landmarks today.

The Emergence of the Laotian Kingdoms (14th to 18th century)

The Laotian people, an ethnic group closely related to the Thais, began to migrate into present-day Laos from southern China during the 8th century. In the 14th century, the Laotian kingdom of Lan Xang emerged as a powerful force in the region. Lan Xang, meaning 'Million Elephants,' was founded by Fa Ngum, a Laotian prince raised at the Khmer court, who unified the principalities under his rule.

Lan Xang experienced a golden age under the reign of King Sisavang Vong, who expanded the kingdom's territory and promoted Buddhism as the state religion.

However, this period of prosperity was followed by a decline due to internal strife and conflicts with neighbouring powers, such as the Burmese and Vietnamese.

In the late 17th century, Lan Xang began fragmenting into smaller kingdoms, including Vientiane, Luang Prabang, and Champasak. These smaller kingdoms were often engaged in conflicts with each other and were vulnerable to invasions from neighbouring powers, such as Siam (now Thailand) and Vietnam.

The Siamese and Vietnamese Dominance (18th to 19th century)

During the 18th century, Laos was caught between two larger expanding regional powers: Siam and Vietnam. Both sought to exert influence and control over the fragmented kingdoms, leading to instability and frequent warfare.

In the early 19th century, Siam emerged as the dominant power in Laos, effectively making the kingdoms its vassal states. However, the Siamese control over Laos was not absolute, and the Lao kingdoms continued to resist Siamese authority throughout the 19th century.

French Protectorate (1893-1953)

As European powers began to colonise Southeast Asia, Laos became a battleground for imperial interests. In 1893, following a series of conflicts between Siam and France, Siam was forced to cede Laos to the French, who incorporated it into their Indochinese empire.

Under French rule, Laos remained a largely rural and neglected backwater. However, the French introduced modern education, built infrastructure, and promoted the cultivation of cash crops such as coffee and rubber. The French also encouraged the growth of Laotian nationalism and fostered a sense of a distinct identity.

During World War II, Laos was occupied by Japanese forces. After the war, France attempted to reassert its control over Laos, but the rise of nationalist and communist movements in the region complicated its efforts. The Laotian Issara (Free Laos) movement, which sought to establish an independent Laos, gained momentum during this period.

The Path to Independence and the Lao Civil War (1953-1975)

In 1953, Laos was granted limited autonomy within the French Union, and full independence was achieved in 1954. However, the country's path to independence was fraught with challenges, including political instability and the emergence of the communist Pathet Laotian movement, which sought to establish a socialist state in Laos.

The Laos Civil War, also known as the Secret War, occurred between 1953 and 1975. It was fought between the Royal Laos Government, backed by the United States, and the communist Pathet Laotian, supported by the Soviet Union, China, and Vietnam. The war was a part of the broader conflict, which included the Vietnam War and the Cambodian Civil War.

During the Laos Civil War, the United States conducted a massive bombing campaign in Laos to disrupt North Vietnamese supply lines and support the Royal Laos Government. The war caused widespread destruction, displaced thousands, and left a legacy of unexploded ordnance that continues to pose a threat today.

Laotian People's Democratic Republic (1975 to present)

In 1975, following the communist victories in Vietnam and Cambodia, the Pathet Laotian emerged victorious in Laos. The monarchy was abolished, and the Laotian People's Democratic Republic was established under the leadership of the Laotian People's Revolutionary Party, which remains the country's sole ruling party.

Since 1975, Laos has pursued a socialist path, maintaining close ties with Vietnam and the Soviet Union during the Cold War. The government implemented collectivisation policies, nationalised industries, and implemented a planned economy. However, these policies stifled economic growth and led to widespread poverty.

In the late 1980s and early 1990s, Laos began implementing market-oriented reforms, opening its economy to foreign investment and gradually shifting towards a more mixed economic system. These reforms have contributed to significant economic growth and development in the country, particularly in the hydropower, mining, and tourism sectors.

Despite its economic progress, Laos continues to face challenges, including poverty, inequality, inadequate infrastructure, and environmental degradation. The country also remains a one-party state with limited political freedoms and human rights concerns.

Throughout its history, Laos has maintained a distinct cultural identity, marked by its Buddhist heritage, traditional arts, and the resilience of its people. As the nation continues to evolve and adapt to the challenges of the modern world, it remains firmly rooted in its rich historical and cultural traditions.

CHAPTER 15
A Brief History Of Cambodia

Population (2023):	17 Million+
Leading religion:	Buddhism
Currency:	Cambodian Riel
Politics and stature:	Constitutional monarchy with a parliamentary system
National sport:	Khmer boxing
Average age:	27
Urbanization:	25 percent
National dish:	Amok trey
National animal:	Kouprey
National plant:	Romduol

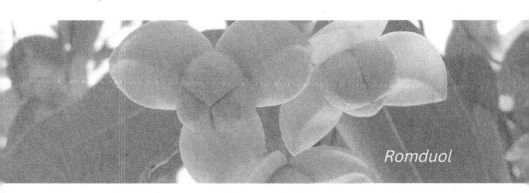

Romduol

Introduction

Nestled in Southeast Asia's heart, Cambodia has a rich and captivating history spanning thousands of years. As a melting pot of various cultures, religions, and political influences, the country has witnessed the rise and fall of mighty empires, legendary kings' reigns, and the indelible impact of foreign forces. This essay delves into the key events, periods and changes that have shaped Cambodia's extraordinary past, offering an insight into the influences that influenced this unique nation.

Prehistoric Cambodia

The story of Cambodia begins in prehistoric times, with archaeological evidence suggesting that the region was inhabited as early as 4000 BCE. The inhabitants of this period were primarily hunters and gatherers, relying on fertile land and abundant natural resources to sustain themselves. It wasn't until the first millennium BCE that rice cultivation and the use of bronze tools began to spread across the region, leading to the establishment of permanent settlements and the formation of early societies.

The Rise of the Funan Kingdom

The first significant political entity in Cambodian history was with the Funan Kingdom, which emerged in the 1st century CE. Influenced by Indian culture and trade, Funan rose to prominence due to its strategic location along the maritime trade routes between India and China. This enabled the kingdom to amass wealth and power, leading to growth and development.

The Funan Kingdom, the 'Land of the Mountain Kings', was a thriving hub of commerce and culture, adopting elements of Hinduism and Buddhism from Indian traders. The kingdom's architecture, art, and administrative systems were heavily influenced by Indian models, resulting in a fascinating fusion of cultures that would lay the foundations for future Cambodian civilisations.

The Flourishing of Chenla

By the 6th century CE, the Funan Kingdom had given way to the emergence of the Chenla Kingdom, which would dominate Cambodia for the next three centuries. Though initially a vassal state of Funan, Chenla eventually absorbed its predecessor and expanded its territory, encompassing present-day Cambodia, Laos and parts of Vietnam.

The Chenla Kingdom adopted Mahayana Buddhism, a shift from the predominantly Hindu Funan period. This transition was mirrored in the kingdom's art and architecture, with many temples featuring both Hindu and Buddhist iconography. The Chenla Kingdom is also notable for its introduction of the Khmer script, which remains the official writing system in Cambodia to this day.

The Golden Age of the Khmer Empire

The true zenith of Cambodia's history came with the emergence of the mighty Khmer Empire, founded by King Jayavarman II in 802 CE. Over the next 600 years, the empire would expand to encompass Cambodia and parts of present-day Thailand, Laos, and Vietnam. The Khmer Empire is synonymous with the classic Angkor period, which saw the construction of the world-famous temple complexes of Angkor Wat and Angkor Thom.

Under the rule of kings such as Suryavarman II and Jayavarman VII, the Khmer Empire thrived, becoming a beacon of art, culture, and architectural innovation. In addition, the empire's hydraulic engineering prowess was showcased in the construction of the vast Baray reservoirs and intricate irrigation systems, which supported a growing population and ensured the success of large-scale agriculture.

However, the decline of the Khmer Empire was inevitable, as internal strife, invasions from neighbouring kingdoms and the gradual erosion of its vast territories took their toll.

By the 15th century, the once-great empire had all but disintegrated, leaving behind a rich architectural legacy that continues to inspire wonder.

The Dark Ages and European Contact

Following the decline of the Khmer Empire, Cambodia entered a long period of fragmentation and turmoil, often referred to as the Dark Ages. The country was plagued by continuous warfare from the 15th to the 19th century as it struggled to defend itself from the encroaching Siamese (Thai) and Vietnamese forces. During this time, the capital shifted multiple times, with the royal court fleeing from Angkor to Phnom Penh in the 15th century, partly due to the increasing threat from the Siamese.

It was during this tumultuous period that Cambodia first encountered European powers. Portuguese and Spanish missionaries, traders and adventurers arrived in the 16th century, establishing diplomatic and trade relations with the beleaguered Cambodian court. The Europeans brought firearms and new technologies, which the Cambodians adopted in their ongoing battles against their regional adversaries.

The French Protectorate

In the 19th century, as European colonial powers expanded their reach across Southeast Asia, Cambodia found itself caught between the territorial ambitions of its neighbours and those of the French. In an attempt to stave off annexation by Siam (Thailand) and Vietnam, King Norodom signed a treaty with the French in 1863, effectively placing Cambodia under French protection. This marked the beginning of the French Protectorate, which would last until 1953.

Under French rule, Cambodia underwent significant modernisation and development, particularly in infrastructure, education and administration. The French were also instrumental in rediscovering and restoring the ancient Angkor temples, which had been largely forgotten since the fall of the Khmer Empire.

However, French colonial rule also imposed cultural and economic domination, leading to growing resentment among the population.

The Struggle for Independence

The seeds of Cambodian nationalism were sown during the French Protectorate, with various nationalist movements emerging throughout the early 20th century. World War II and the Japanese occupation of Cambodia further weakened French control, paving the way for the push for independence.

In 1953, under the leadership of King Norodom Sihanouk, Cambodia successfully negotiated its independence from France, signalling the end of colonial rule and the beginning of a new era for the nation. Sihanouk abdicated the throne in 1955 but remained a pivotal figure in Cambodian politics as head of state, steering the country through a period of relative stability and neutrality during the early years of the Cold War.

The Khmer Rouge and the Cambodian Genocide

The late 1960s and 1970s marked a dark chapter in Cambodia's history as the country became embroiled in the broader conflict in Indochina. With the escalation of the Vietnam War, Cambodia was increasingly drawn into the conflict, culminating in the rise of the brutal Khmer Rouge regime under Pol Pot in 1975.

The Khmer Rouge's radical communist policies forced millions of Cambodians to rural labour camps, where countless people perished from starvation, disease and execution. It is estimated that between 1.7 and 2 million Cambodians – around a quarter of the population – lost their lives during the four-year rule of the Khmer Rouge.

Recovery and Reconciliation

The Khmer Rouge was toppled in 1979 by Vietnamese forces, which installed a new, more moderate government in Cambodia. The country then embarked on a long and arduous journey of recovery and reconciliation, grappling with the immense trauma and devastation.

Cambodia has made strides in rebuilding its society, economy and political structures in the following decades.

Cambodia Today: Progress and Challenges

In the 21st century, Cambodia has experienced remarkable economic growth, fuelled by a booming tourism industry, increased foreign investment, and the development of the manufacturing sector. The country has made great strides in reducing poverty, improving healthcare, and expanding educational opportunities for its people.

The Cambodian government has tried to promote sustainable development and preserve the nation's rich cultural heritage. For example, the protection and restoration of the Angkor temple complex have become a symbol of national pride and identity, attracting millions of visitors each year.

The history of Cambodia is a fascinating tapestry of triumphs and tragedies, a testament to the resilience and spirit of its people. From the heights of the Khmer Empire to the depths of the Khmer Rouge's terror, Cambodia has emerged as a nation determined to learn from its past and forge a brighter future. As the country continues to evolve and progress, its rich history serves as a poignant reminder of the indomitable spirit that has carried Cambodia through the ages.

CHAPTER 16

A Brief History Of Vietnam

Population (2023):	99 Million+
Leading religion:	Buddhism
Currency:	Vietnamese Dong
Politics and stature:	Communist Party of Vietnam (CPV), a single-party socialist republic
National sport:	Da cau
Average age:	32
Urbanization:	37 percent
National dish:	Pho
National animal:	Buffalo
National plant:	Lotus Flower

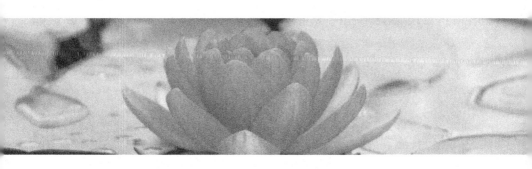

Introduction

The history of Vietnam, a country nestled along the eastern coast of the Indochinese Peninsula in Southeast Asia, is a rich tapestry of culture, conflict, and resilience. From the ancient kingdoms of the Red River Delta to the challenges of the modern era, the story of Vietnam is marked by adversity and triumph. This overview of Vietnamese history explores the key events and milestones that have shaped the nation from its earliest beginnings to the present day.

Early Civilisations and Chinese Rule

The history of Vietnam can be traced back to the Bronze Age cultures of the Dong Son and Sa Huynh, which flourished in the Red River Delta and central Vietnam, respectively. These early civilisations were characterised by their unique artistic traditions, particularly the intricate bronze drum craftsmanship of the Dong Son culture.

In 111 BC, the Chinese Han Dynasty annexed the Red River Delta, marking the beginning of a millennium of Chinese rule over the region. Under Chinese domination, Vietnam, then known as Nam Viet, underwent a process of sinicization, adopting the Chinese language, political systems, and Confucian values. This period also saw the rise of several notable Vietnamese resistance movements, including the Trung Sisters' rebellion in 40 AD and the Ly Nam De uprising in 542 AD, which sought to restore Vietnamese independence.

The Ly, Tran, and Le Dynasties

Vietnamese independence was finally achieved in 939 AD when Ngo Quyen defeated the Chinese at the Battle of Bach Dang River, establishing the Ngo Dynasty. This victory began a long period of Vietnamese self-rule, characterised by establishing several powerful dynasties.

The Ly Dynasty (1009-1225) marked a period of significant cultural and political development, with the founding of the Vietnamese capital, Thang Long (modern-day Hanoi), and the emergence of a strong centralised government. The Ly Dynasty was also known for supporting Buddhism, which became the state religion during this period.

The Tran Dynasty (1225-1400) succeeded the Ly Dynasty and continued to strengthen the Vietnamese state through territorial expansion and political reforms. However, the Tran Dynasty is best known for its military victories against the Mongol invasions in 1258, 1285, and 1288, cemented Vietnam's status as a formidable regional power.

The Le Dynasty (1428-1788) was founded by Le Loi after a successful rebellion against Chinese rule, marking another period of prosperity and cultural achievement in Vietnam. Under the reign of Emperor Le Thanh Tong, the country experienced a golden age of literature, art, and education, culminating in the creation of the Quoc Ngu, the modern Vietnamese script based on the Latin alphabet.

The Tay Son Rebellion and the Nguyen Dynasty

The 18th century saw internal conflict and chaos in Vietnam, known as the Tay Son Rebellion (1771-1802). This peasant-led uprising sought to overthrow the ruling Le and Nguyen lords, ultimately leading to the temporary unification of Vietnam under the Tay Son brothers.

The Tay Son rule was short-lived, however, as Nguyen Anh, a surviving member of the Nguyen family, enlisted the support of French missionaries and the French navy to regain control of Vietnam. In 1802, Nguyen Anh defeated the Tay Son forces and established the Nguyen Dynasty, the last of Vietnam's royal dynasties. He took the name Gia Long and founded the capital in Hue, centralising his rule over a unified Vietnam.

French Colonisation and Indochina

The 19th century marked the beginning of French involvement in Vietnam, as France sought to expand its colonial empire in Southeast Asia. After a series of military campaigns and diplomatic manoeuvres, France established control over Vietnam, Cambodia, and Laos, forming the colony of French Indochina in 1887. Under French rule, Vietnam underwent significant social, economic, and political changes, with the introduction of Western education, infrastructure, and legal systems.

Despite the modernisation brought about by French colonisation, the Vietnamese faced widespread discrimination, exploitation, and loss of political autonomy. These conditions fuelled the rise of several nationalist movements, which sought to resist French rule and restore Vietnamese sovereignty. Among these movements was the Indochinese Communist Party, founded by Ho Chi Minh in 1930, which would later play a pivotal role in Vietnam's struggle for independence.

World War II and the First Indochina War

During World War II, Japan occupied Vietnam and used the country as a base for its military operations in Southeast Asia. The Japanese occupation further weakened French control over Vietnam, allowing nationalist movements to gain momentum.

Following Japan's surrender in 1945, Ho Chi Minh declared Vietnam's independence, establishing the Democratic Republic of Vietnam (DRV) in the north. However, France refused to recognise the DRV and sought to regain control over its former colony, leading to the outbreak of the First Indochina War (1946-1954).

The war culminated in the decisive Battle of Dien Bien Phu, where the Vietnamese forces, led by General Vo Nguyen Giap, defeated the French colonial army.

This victory marked the end of French rule in Vietnam. It led to the signing of the Geneva Accords in 1954, temporarily dividing Vietnam along the 17th parallel, with the communist DRV in the north and the non-communist State of Vietnam, backed by the United States, in the south.

The Vietnam War and Reunification

The division of Vietnam set the stage for the Vietnam War (1955-1975). This conflict pitted the communist government of North Vietnam and its southern allies, the Viet Cong, against the government of South Vietnam and its main ally, the United States. The war was characterised by widespread violence, guerrilla warfare tactics, and the deployment of controversial strategies, such as Agent Orange, by the United States.

In 1973, following years of mounting anti-war sentiment and the signing of the Paris Peace Accords, the United States withdrew its troops from Vietnam, leaving the South Vietnamese government to face the advancing North Vietnamese forces alone. In 1975, North Vietnam captured the southern capital, Saigon, effectively ending the war and reunifying the country under communist rule.

Post-War Vietnam and the Doi Moi Reforms

Following the end of the Vietnam War, the country faced significant challenges, including widespread poverty, economic stagnation, and international isolation. In response to these challenges, the Vietnamese government launched a series of economic and political reforms in 1986, known as the Doi Moi ('Renovation') policy. These reforms aimed to transform Vietnam's centrally planned economy into a socialist-oriented market economy while maintaining the country's one-party communist system.

The Doi Moi reforms have had a transformative impact on Vietnam, leading to significant economic growth, increased foreign investment, and the gradual integration of the country into the global economy.

Vietnam is recognised as one of the world's fastest-growing economies and a key player in Southeast Asia's regional politics and security. The history of Vietnam is a story of resilience, resistance, and adaptation. From the ancient civilisations of the Red River Delta to the challenges of the modern era, the Vietnamese people have navigated a complex and tumultuous past to emerge as a strong and dynamic nation in the 21st century. This rich historical tapestry provides valuable insight into the complex cultural, political, and social forces that have shaped Vietnam and its people over the centuries.

NOTES

NOTES

Printed in Great Britain
by Amazon

46328970R00129